NUTRITION AND FITNESS

4

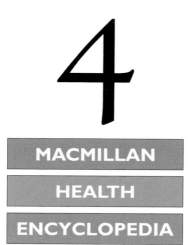

MACMILLAN

HEALTH

ENCYCLOPEDIA

NUTRITION AND FITNESS

4

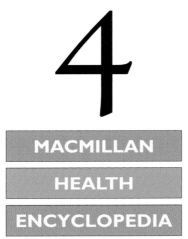

MACMILLAN

HEALTH

ENCYCLOPEDIA

MACMILLAN REFERENCE USA

EDITORIAL CREDITS

Developed and produced by
Visual Education Corporation, Princeton, NJ
Project Editor: Cynthia E. Mooney
Editor: Amy Livingston
Associate Editor: Eleanor R. Hero
Photo Editor: Sara Matthews
Production Supervisor: William A. Murray
Copyediting Supervisor: Maureen Ryan Pancza
Art Editor: Christine Osborne
Advisors, Anatomical Illustrations:
John A. Negulesco, Ph.D.
Department of Biology, Neurobiology, and Anatomy
The Ohio State University, College of Medicine
Columbus, OH

David Seiden, Ph.D.
Robert Wood Johnson Medical School
Piscataway, NJ
Electronic Production: Kathleen Caratozzolo,
     Lisa Evans-Skopas, Isabelle Ulsh
Electronic Preparation: Cynthia Feldner, Fiona Torphy
Design: Hespenheide Design

The information contained in the *Macmillan Health Encyclopedia* is not intended to take the place of the care and advice of a physician or healthcare professional. Readers should obtain professional advice in making health care decisions.

PHOTO CREDITS

© Corbis: 118

© Tom Dunham: 12, 19, 22, 25 (both), 40, 46, 60, 72, 81, 82, 101 (bottom), 103, 112, 114 (right), 116, 121, 122, 125, 126, 127, 128, 133

© F-Stock Photo Agency: John Laptad, 101 (top); Caroline Wood, 113

© George White Location Photography: 38

© Index Stock Imagery: Kindra Clineff, 100

© inStock: Philip Slagter, 78

© Leo de Wys, Inc.: Alan Dolgins, 90

© David Madison: 5, 7, 28 (top), 77, 131, 132; Shelby Thorner, 10 (right)

© Photo Researchers, Inc.: Rafael Macia, 141; Fred J. Maroon, 71 (top); Sam Ogden/Science Photo Library, 48 (bottom); Charles D. Winters/Timeframe Photography, Inc., 20

© PhotoEdit: Vic Bider, 59 (top); Robert Brenner, 29, 48 (top); Jose Carrillo, 28 (bottom); Myrleen Ferguson Cate, 21, 62, 93; Tony Freeman, 39, 51, 76, 98; Spencer Grant, 57; Felicia Martinez, 50, 54, 95; Tom McCarthy, 4, 44; Michael Newman, 30, 69 (top), 139; Alan Oddie, 17 (right); Tom Prettyman, 10 (left); Susan Van Etten, 119; David Young-Wolff, 13, 58, 91, 115, 134

© SGM Photography: Robert Matthews, 9, 33, 34, 35, 49, 59 (bottom), 66, 69 (bottom)

© Unicorn Stock Photos: Steve Bourgeois, 56; Jay Foreman, 17 (left); Martha McBride, 114 (left); Tom McCarthy, 110

USDA-ARS Information Staff: 71 (bottom)

Macmillan Library Reference USA
1633 Broadway
New York, NY 10019-6785

Printed in the United States of America

printing number
10 9 8 7 6 5 4 3 2 1

Library of Congress Cataloging-in-Publication Data
Macmillan health encyclopedia.
     p.   cm.
     Includes bibliographical references and index.
     Contents: v. 1. Body systems—v. 2. Communicable diseases—v. 3. Noncommunicable diseases and disorders—v. 4. Nutrition and fitness—v. 5. Emotional and mental health—v. 6. Sexuality and reproduction—v. 7. Drugs, alcohol, and tobacco—v. 8. Safety and environmental health—v. 9. Health care systems, cumulative index.
     ISBN 0-02-865036-0 (set).—ISBN 0-02-865040-9 (v. 1).—ISBN 0-02-865041-7 (v. 2)
     1. Health Encyclopedias.   I. Macmillan Reference USA.
RA776.M174   1999
610'.3—dc21   99-23432
                                                        CIP

Volumes of the *Macmillan Health Encyclopedia*

1 *Body Systems* (ISBN 0-02-865040-9)
2 *Communicable Diseases* (ISBN 0-02-865041-7)
3 *Noncommunicable Diseases and Disorders* (ISBN 0-02-865042-5)
4 *Nutrition and Fitness* (ISBN 0-02-865043-3)
5 *Emotional and Mental Health* (ISBN 0-02-865044-1)
6 *Sexuality and Reproduction* (ISBN 0-02-865045-X)
7 *Drugs, Alcohol, and Tobacco* (ISBN 0-02-865046-8)
8 *Safety and Environmental Health* (ISBN 0-02-865047-6)
9 *Health Care Systems/Cumulative Index* (ISBN 0-02-865048-4)

PREFACE

The *Macmillan Health Encyclopedia* is a nine-volume set that explains how the body works; describes the causes and treatment of hundreds of diseases and disorders; provides information on diet and exercise for a healthy lifestyle; discusses key issues in emotional, mental, and sexual health; covers problems related to the use and abuse of legal and illegal drugs; outlines first-aid procedures; and provides up-to-date information on current health issues.

Written with the support of a distinguished panel of editorial advisors, the encyclopedia puts considerable emphasis on the idea of wellness. It discusses measures an individual can take to prevent illness and provides information about healthy lifestyle choices.

The *Macmillan Health Encyclopedia* is organized topically. Each of the nine volumes relates to an area covered in the school health curriculum. The encyclopedia also supplements course work in biology, psychology, home economics, and physical education. The volumes are organized as follows: 1. *Body Systems: Anatomy and Physiology;* 2. *Communicable Diseases: Symptoms, Diagnosis, Treatment;* 3. *Noncommunicable Diseases and Disorders: Symptoms, Diagnosis, Treatment;* 4. *Nutrition and Fitness;* 5. *Emotional and Mental Health;* 6. *Sexuality and Reproduction;* 7. *Drugs, Alcohol, and Tobacco;* 8. *Safety and Environmental Health;* 9. *Health Care Systems/Cumulative Index.*

The information in the *Macmillan Health Encyclopedia* is clearly presented and easy to find. Entries are arranged in alphabetical order within each volume. An extensive system of cross-referencing directs the reader from a synonym to the main entry (GERMAN MEASLES see RUBELLA) and from one entry to additional information in other entries. Words printed in SMALL CAPITALS ("These substances, found in a number of NONPRESCRIPTION DRUGS . . .") indicate that there is an entry of that name in the volume. Most entries end with a list of "see also" cross-references to related topics. Entries within the same volume have no number (See also ANTI-INFLAMMATORY DRUGS); entries located in another volume include the volume number (See also HYPERTENSION, 3). All topics covered in a volume can be found in the index at the back of the book. There is also a cumulative index to the set in Volume 9.

The extensive use of illustration includes colorful drawings, photographs, charts, and graphs to supplement and enrich the information presented in the text. Questions of particular concern to the reader—When should I see a doctor? What are the risk factors? What can I do to prevent an illness?—are indicated by the following marginal notations: Consult a Physician, Risk Factors, and Healthy Choices.

Each volume of the encyclopedia also has its own GLOSSARY. Located in the front of the book, the glossary provides brief definitions of medical or technical terms with which the reader may not be familiar. Difficult terms that are not included in the glossary are explained within the context of the entry. Such terms are set in *italic* type. *Italic* type is also used for terms that are not entry titles, but on which the reader will find helpful information elsewhere in the encyclopedia. The special type reminds the reader to check the cumulative index to locate more information.

A SUPPLEMENTARY SOURCES section at the back of the book contains a listing of suggested reading material as well as organizations from which additional information can be obtained.

GLOSSARY

acid-base balance The balance maintained by the body between too much and too little acid in body fluids.

addiction Physical or psychological dependence on chemical substances such as alcohol or other drugs; any habit so strong that it cannot be given up easily.

allergy An oversensitivity of the immune system to certain substances (such as foods, chemicals, pollens, and insect bites) that causes formation of antibodies.

amino acids A group of chemical compounds that form the basic structure of proteins. There are nine essential amino acids.

antibody A chemical substance produced by the body in response to invading microorganisms, such as bacteria or viruses. An antibody neutralizes or destroys the foreign organism.

antioxidant A chemical compound that prevents oxygen from reacting with other compounds.

autoimmune Pertains to disorders caused by the reaction of an individual's immune system to the body's own tissue. The body reacts by producing antibodies, the same way it would react to an invading organism.

bacteria (sing. *bacterium*) Single-celled, microscopic organisms, abundant in living things, air, soil, and water. Some are beneficial to humans, while others cause disease (see MICRO-ORGANISMS, **2**).

blood pressure The force exerted by blood against the walls of arteries. It is measured when the heart contracts and when it relaxes between contractions.

blood sugar level The concentration of glucose in the bloodstream.

cardiovascular endurance The ability of the heart, lungs, and blood vessels to carry enough oxygen to function efficiently during an extended period of vigorous movement.

catalyst A substance that speeds up a chemical reaction without being changed or destroyed by the reaction.

colostrum Thick, yellowish fluid, rich in antibodies and other protective factors, produced by the mother's breast in the first 2 to 3 days after the birth of a baby. It is then replaced by breast milk.

communicable Refers to disease caused by microorganisms or parasites that can be transmitted from one person or animal to another.

constipation A condition in which bowels are not emptied easily or often enough.

contagious Refers to the time period when an infected person is able to pass an infectious disease to another person by direct or indirect contact; also used to describe the person who can spread the disease.

edema Any swelling of the body caused by an abnormal accumulation of fluid in spaces between tissues, organs, or cells.

enzyme A type of protein, produced in the cells, that causes specific chemical processes to take place in the body. Some enzymes, for example, help break down food.

feces Solid waste material eliminated from the body.

fluoride A mineral useful in helping to prevent tooth decay. It is thought to increase the mineral content of tooth enamel and make it more resistant to the acid in foods.

fortified Refers to the addition of one or more nutrients to a food item that is not normally a good source of the nutrient, such as vitamin D to milk, calcium to orange juice, or certain vitamins to cereals.

gastrointestinal tract The part of the digestive system consisting of the mouth, esophagus, stomach, and intestines, but excluding the liver, gallbladder, and pancreas.

genes Structures in cells that are inherited from parents; important in determining an individual's physical and mental characteristics.

glucagon   A hormone, formed in the pancreas, that causes the release of stored glucose.

glycogen   The principle substance for storing carbohydrates in the body. Glycogen is stored in the liver and muscle tissue, changed into glucose, and released into the bloodstream when blood sugar levels fall.

hemoglobin   Protein that contains iron and is found in red blood cells; transports oxygen from the lungs to the body.

hereditary   Passed down from parents to children by means of genes.

hormone   A chemical substance, such as insulin or estrogen, that stimulates and regulates certain bodily functions.

hypertension   High blood pressure.

infection   A condition caused by bacteria, viruses, fungi, or other microorganisms that invade and damage body cells and tissues.

inorganic   Made up of or pertaining to matter that is neither animal nor vegetable; not involving living organisms.

insoluble   Impossible to dissolve.

insulin   A hormone, secreted by certain cells of the pancreas, that helps the body use sugars and starches.

legume   A plant with seeds growing in pods, such as peas, beans, or lentils.

lymphatic system   Part of the immune system; a loosely organized system of vessels and ducts that carry lymph fluid from the spaces between cells into the bloodstream.

macromineral   Any mineral needed and used by the body in relatively large amounts, such as calcium, potassium, or sodium.

macronutrient   Any nutrient that the body needs continually in large amounts for essential function: for example, protein, carbohydrates, or fats.

metabolism   The physical and chemical processes of the body that convert food into energy and body tissue.

micromineral   Any mineral needed and used by the body in very small amounts, such as iron or zinc.

micronutrient   A nutrient that the body needs in very small amounts for essential functions.

net weight   The weight of a packaged food item, exclusive of the weight of the packaging.

opiate   Any narcotic pain reliever, such as morphine, heroin, or opium.

organic   Pertains to living organisms (plants and animals). Also used to describe a food or nutrient produced without the use of chemical fertilizers, pesticides, or additives.

oxidize   To unite with oxygen.

pH balance   The acidity or alkalinity of a substance; the letters stand for "potential of Hydrogen."

physiological   Pertaining to the processes, activities, and functions of the body.

processed food   Any food that has been altered in texture, mixed with additives, or cooked.

soluble   Able to be dissolved.

toxicity   The property of being poisonous; the severity of the adverse effects or illness produced by a toxin.

tuber   The thick, fleshy part of an underground stem.

vascular   Pertaining to the blood vessels and the circulation of blood.

virus   Very small infectious agent that requires a living cell in order to reproduce (see MICROORGANISMS, **2**).

▶ AEROBIC DANCE

Aerobic dance includes AEROBIC EXERCISE routines that use rhythmic movements set to music to improve respiratory and circulatory function. Aerobic dance can be an excellent way to burn calories and improve *cardiovascular fitness*. One hour of continuous aerobic dancing can burn as much as 600 calories. Aerobic dancing also improves FLEXIBILITY, coordination, and, to a lesser degree, STRENGTH.

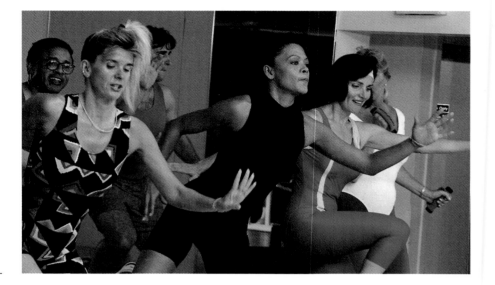

Aerobic Dance Class. *One of the advantages of aerobic dance for many people is that it enables them to exercise in a social setting.*

How It Is Done Aerobic dance is a popular form of EXERCISE, particularly among women. It is typically performed two to three times a week, often in a group led by an instructor. A session usually consists of 5 to 10 minutes of gradual warm-up, followed by 20 to 50 minutes of vigorous exercise, ending with a 5- to 10-minute cooldown. People who cannot attend an aerobics class may purchase videotapes to follow at home.

Aerobic Dance Safety If you decide to enter an aerobic dance program, choose one with a duration and intensity that match your level of FITNESS. Other factors to consider include the qualifications of the instructor, the hardness of the floor, the frequency of class meetings, and the WARM-UP AND COOLDOWN practices. Be sure to wear supportive, well-cushioned shoes that fit well, and avoid jarring motions. Aerobic dance must be performed regularly to promote fitness. A workout that lasts at least 30 minutes and is repeated at least three times a week is recommended for improving cardiovascular health. (See also ENDURANCE; FITNESS TRAINING; HEART RATE.)

▶ AEROBIC EXERCISE

Aerobic exercise is continuous EXERCISE that can be sustained for long periods of time without causing exhaustion. Examples include RUNNING, WALKING, CYCLING, and SWIMMING. These differ from other energetic activities such as football and gymnastics, which involve periods of effort followed by slack periods during which the body can recover. ANAEROBIC EXERCISES, such as sprinting, are also distinct. They involve muscular effort so intense that energy is used faster than the body can produce it. Anaerobic exercise cannot be sustained.

The Benefits of Aerobic Exercise Aerobic exercise can provide several health benefits. For example, it is the key to cardiovascular fitness, one of the most important components of physical health. *Cardiovascular fitness* means having a strong heart, efficient lungs, and an effective circulatory system.

Regular aerobic workouts increase the strength of the heart muscle so that it can pump more blood with each contraction (beat). This means that although the heart rate still increases during exercise, the average heart rate is lower, putting less strain on your system. The heart does less work to achieve the same level of activity and recovers from the stress of exercise more quickly, returning to the resting heart rate in a shorter period of time.

Regular aerobic exercise helps the lungs function better. The amount of air they can take in and breathe out at one time increases. In addition, the muscles develop a more extensive network of blood vessels. This allows the blood to transport oxygen and NUTRIENTS more efficiently to the heart muscle as well as to other muscles of the body.

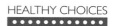

Aerobic exercise has other important health benefits. It can help keep blood pressure at normal levels and help control weight. It may also raise the blood levels of HDL CHOLESTEROL (the "good" cholesterol) and lower blood sugar levels. Active, fit people have a considerably lower death rate from heart disease and cancer than do people who are unfit. Fit people also have a lower risk of developing other diseases such as Type 2 (non-insulin-dependent) diabetes and osteoporosis. Regular aerobic exercise may have psychological benefits as well, including improved self-esteem, reduced anxiety and depression, and an increased ability to deal with stress.

The Limitations of Aerobic Exercise Although aerobic exercise improves the efficiency of the cardiovascular system, it does not necessarily promote the other components of overall FITNESS, particularly STRENGTH and FLEXIBILITY. For example, many aerobic activities, such as running and cycling, do little to increase muscle strength and endurance in the upper body.

Aerobic Exercise. *Aerobic exercise promotes cardiovascular health, an important part of fitness.*

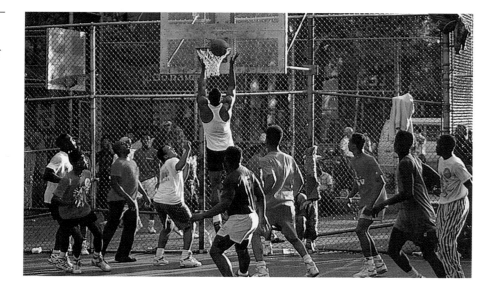

To achieve overall fitness, you should supplement aerobic activities with STRENGTH TRAINING exercises at least two to three times a week. An efficient way to improve flexibility is to include STRETCHING EXERCISES in each aerobic workout.

How to Achieve Aerobic Conditioning   Any exercise that raises your heart rate and keeps it there for a prolonged time—at least 20 minutes—will help you achieve aerobic conditioning. Many vigorous sports and activities that fit this description include AEROBIC DANCE, rope jumping, rowing, cross-country skiing, and racquetball. People with back or knee problems can participate in a type of aerobic activity called *low-impact aerobics* that jars the body less. Low-impact aerobic activities include racewalking, swimming, and special low-impact dance and exercise routines. A habit of regular brisk walking improves aerobic fitness and provides most of the health benefits of more strenuous programs.

Any amount of aerobic exercise is good for your health and fitness, but to achieve the maximum health benefit, most experts recommend that aerobic exercise be performed continuously for a minimum of 20 to 30 minutes, three times a week. To increase conditioning or speed weight loss, a person should exercise more frequently and for longer periods. Hard workouts should be alternated each day with less demanding sessions to prevent muscle strain.

To promote optimum cardiovascular fitness through aerobic exercise, try to maintain your HEART RATE within a target range: from 60 to 80 percent of your maximum heart rate (which can be estimated as 220 minus your age in years). You should check your pulse several times during an aerobic exercise session to make sure that your heart rate is within these limits.

Aerobic exercise should be preceded by a warm-up period, 5 to 10 minutes of low intensity exercise designed to increase blood flow to working muscles. This prepares your body for more vigorous exercise. Every session should end with a cooldown, a time of light activity, to let the heart rate gradually return to normal. If you neglect the cooldown, you may feel light-headed or dizzy.

Anyone participating in strenuous physical activity should be alert to signs that suggest the activity be discontinued. Stop exercising if symptoms such as unusual breathlessness, nausea, or dizziness occur. Acute chest pain or pressure, or pain radiating through the shoulder or arm for more than 2 minutes, may be very serious; if these symptoms occur, medical help should be summoned immediately. (See also ENDURANCE; FITNESS TRAINING; SPORTS AND FITNESS; WARM-UP AND COOLDOWN.)

► **AGRICULTURAL CHEMICALS**   Agricultural chemicals are substances used by farmers to improve the quantity and quality of the foods they produce. These chemicals work in a variety of ways and include fertilizers, pesticides, and growth regulators.

Fertilizers   Fertilizers are used to provide plants with essential nutrients for growth. "Organic" fertilizers consist of decomposed plant material and manure. "Chemical" fertilizers are usually manufactured, primarily in the form of inorganic salts. Both types of fertilizers deliver the same basic nutrients to the soil.

Pesticides   Pesticides are chemicals that are applied to crops to control insects, fungi, rodents, and competing plants and weeds. Pesticides are poisons: The *-cide* ending means "killer." Ideally, they should do their job and then break down into harmless substances before the food is eaten. In reality, traces of pesticides can remain on fruits and vegetables all the way to the consumer's table. The Food and Drug Administration (FDA) recently passed new regulations that require manufacturers to show that there is a "reasonable certainty of no harm" from consuming foods grown with pesticides. These new standards protect infants and young children, who have a greater risk of becoming sick from pesticide residues than adults do. Although the amounts of pesticide found in food should not be dangerous, you should still wash all produce before eating it.

Growth Regulators   Growth regulators are used to enhance the growth and size of both plants and animals. They do so by artificially mimicking natural substances called *hormones.* In plants, they typically have no residual effect on the resulting food products. Their use in meat production, however, is considerably more controversial. Although studies have shown that meat and milk from cows treated with hormones are safe, many people feel that the use of these hormones affects the quality of these foods. Controlled use of growth stimulants is currently allowed in meats and poultry marketed in the United States but is prohibited in many European countries. (See also FOOD ADDITIVES; FOOD SAFETY.)

▶ ANAEROBIC EXERCISE

Anaerobic exercise is exercise that causes the body to incur an *oxygen debt,* in which the muscles have used up the oxygen supply and are working without oxygen. It is intense EXERCISE, such as weight lifting or sprinting, that lasts for only a short period of time. Whenever the cells' supply of energy is used up faster than the heart and lungs can provide them with oxygen to make more energy, the body must instead rely on energy from carbohydrates that are stored in the bloodstream as GLUCOSE and in the muscles as *glycogen.*

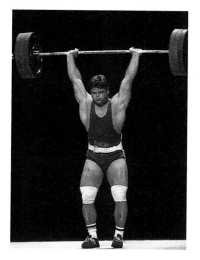

Anaerobic Exercise. *Trained as well as untrained individuals may experience uncomfortable symptoms immediately after strenuous anaerobic exercise.*

Effects of Anaerobic Exercise   Because anaerobic exercise uses up the muscles' oxygen supply, *lactic acid* (a by-product of muscle use) builds up in the muscles. For the muscles to return to normal, the lactic acid must combine with new oxygen when the exercise is over. After an anaerobic activity, most people continue to breathe deeply and rapidly in order to get more oxygen to the muscle cells that need it. Extreme anaerobic activity may also produce headache, blurry vision, nausea, vomiting, or light-headedness. These symptoms result from a buildup of lactic acid and, although uncomfortable, are not serious. When they occur, the person should keep moving or walking until they subside. Although most people feel better within a few minutes, full recovery can take 1 to 2 hours, depending on the extent of the lactic acid buildup.

The Role of Anaerobic Exercise in a Fitness Program   Many forms of anaerobic exercise are too intense for people who are just starting a fitness program. AEROBIC EXERCISE is a better choice for them because it puts less stress on the body while improving cardiovascular health. However, anaerobic exercise can be an important part of a fitness program if the heart and circulatory system are already well conditioned. This type of exercise can help develop STRENGTH together with muscular and cardiovascular ENDURANCE. Weight lifting, for example, helps develop strong muscles. Over time, anaerobic exercise will increase the efficiency with which the cells use oxygen, resulting in improved performance during aerobic exercise. (See also BODYBUILDING; FITNESS; FITNESS TRAINING; STRENGTH TRAINING.)

▶ ANOREXIA NERVOSA   see EATING DISORDERS

▶ APPETITE

Appetite is a healthy desire for food. It is the pleasant sensation people feel in anticipation of eating.

Appetite should not be confused with hunger. Appetite is a learned response; HUNGER is a physiological response to the need for food. Hunger is often unpleasant and sometimes painful. The feelings of appetite, hunger, and *satiety* (feeling full) work together to regulate eating behaviors in ways that are not fully understood.

Both physical and psychological factors can cause people to lose their appetite. Illness or emotional upset may cause a temporary loss of appetite. Psychological disorders, such as depression, sometimes result in a persistent loss of appetite. For example, *anorexia nervosa,* a serious psychological condition marked by an irrational fear of gaining weight, causes a suppression of appetite.

The appetite can also increase for physical and psychological reasons. For instance, an *overactive thyroid gland* increases energy requirements and stimulates a person's appetite. The smell, taste, or appearance of food may also spur a person's appetite, as may an increased level of exercise.

Some people use drugs called *appetite suppressants* to lose weight. These drugs work by decreasing a person's appetite; they should be used only for a short time and always under a physician's supervision. Long-term use is generally not an effective means of weight loss and may lead to addiction. Prolonged use can also cause dangerous side effects such as heart and nervous system problems. Two appetite suppressant drugs were recently banned by the Food and Drug Administration (FDA) because they caused depression, heart valve disorders, and a rare and often deadly lung disease. The FDA has also proposed warning labels on products that contain *ephedrine,* a natural herbal extract that acts as an appetite suppressant and can overstimulate the heart and nervous system. (See also DIETS; EATING DISORDERS; FOOD CRAVING; HUNGER; WEIGHT MANAGEMENT; THYROID DISORDERS, 3; ANOREXIA/BULIMIA, 5.)

► ARTIFICIAL SWEETENERS

Artificial sweeteners are synthetic substances used in place of SUGAR to sweeten foods and drinks. They are found in powdered table-sugar substitutes and in processed foods and drinks. Artificial sweeteners taste like sugar but have few or no CALORIES, so they are popular with people who are dieting to lose weight. However, they have little or no nutritional value. The three best-known artificial sweeteners are *saccharin, cyclamate,* and *aspartame.*

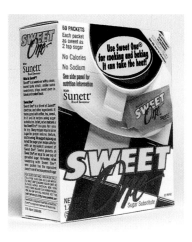

Artificial Sweeteners. *Artificial sweeteners are used in place of table sugar and appear as ingredients in some foods.*

Saccharin, first introduced at the end of the nineteenth century, is used as an ingredient in some products and as a powdered sugar substitute. In the late 1970s, its safety was challenged because scientists identified a possible link between saccharin consumption and tumors in laboratory rats. Although the Food and Drug Administration (FDA) considered banning the product, extensive studies have failed to demonstrate that saccharin causes cancer in humans. In the United States, however, all products containing saccharin must now include a warning label. Its use is banned in Canada, except by prescription.

Cyclamate, introduced in the 1950s, was widely used as a sweetener until 1970, when it was banned from the American market because of a possible link to cancer in laboratory animals. However, more recent studies have shown that this sweetener is unlikely to be harmful to humans. Its use remains legal in Canada.

Aspartame, introduced in 1981 and known most commonly to consumers as NutraSweet, is used in soft drinks, chewing gum, and cereal, among other foods. It is also used in some powdered sugar substitutes. Roughly 200 times as sweet as *sucrose,* or table sugar, aspartame results from the chemical marriage of two amino acids, neither of which is sweet by itself. One of these two amino acids can be dangerous to people who suffer from a rare disorder called phenylketonuria (PKU), and therefore products containing aspartame must carry a warning label. For most people, however, aspartame is considered safe in the amounts normally consumed. Today it is by far the most popular artificial sweetener in the United States.

Two new artificial sweeteners were approved by the FDA in 1998. Acesulfame-K (Sunett) is 200 times as sweet as sugar. When mixed with aspartame, it produces a more sugarlike flavor without an aftertaste. Sucralose (Splenda) is an artificial sweetener made from sugar. A minor chemical change makes sucralose calorie free and 600 times as sweet as sugar. Unlike other sweeteners, it is unlikely to break down at high temperatures, so it can be used for more methods of cooking and baking. Both new sweeteners are considered safe and do not require warning labels. (See also DIET FOOD.)

► ATHLETIC FOOTWEAR

Athletic footwear includes all shoes that are specially constructed to protect the foot and maximize performance in sports activities. Today, people can choose from many kinds of athletic footwear designed for specific sports, including RUNNING, tennis, basketball, aerobics, and WALKING.

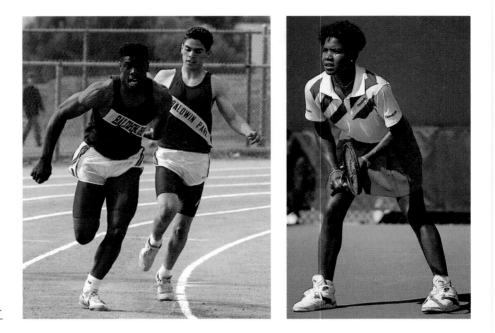

Proper Footwear. *Sports that involve mostly forward motion (such as running) require different footwear than do sports that involve stops, starts, and sideways movements (such as tennis).*

Types of Footwear Athletic footwear differs in the thickness and rigidity of the shoe's sole, the height of the ankle collar, the amount and placement of cushioning, the construction of the heel, and a variety of other features, depending on the sport for which it is intended. In general, however, there are two classes of athletic footwear. One type is designed for activities that involve primarily forward motion, such as running and walking. The second type is for activities that involve a lot of sudden stopping, starting, and lateral motion, such as tennis and aerobic dance: These shoes are reinforced under the toe and have sturdier sides than do running shoes. As a result, they also tend to be a bit heavier.

Orthotic Devices When some people run, their feet tend to roll inward (*pronation*) or outward (*supination*), putting additional stress on the knees, hips, back, and ankles. When the rolling is severe or causes recurring pain, doctors who specialize in foot problems may prescribe orthotic devices, or orthoses. These custom-made devices of foam, leather, or plastic fit inside the wearer's running shoes. Orthotic devices correct improper foot motion and make sports activities easier and more comfortable. They may also be used to relieve other foot problems.

Purchasing Footwear It is not necessary to purchase a separate pair of athletic shoes for each kind of sports activity. Running shoes are best for running, but tennis or basketball shoes can be worn for many other kinds of sports, including aerobic dance, racquetball, and volleyball. Many people find that high-topped shoes support the ankle and prevent the foot from rolling over.

Athletic shoes can be expensive and should be chosen with care to prevent discomfort and injury. Choose footwear that fits well and feels comfortable. Even top-quality athletic shoes lose their ability to absorb shock over time. Replace shoes when they become worn.

▶ BALANCED DIET

HEALTHY CHOICES
■●●●●●●●●●●●●

A balanced diet is an eating plan that includes enough foods from all five basic food groups of the FOOD GUIDE PYRAMID to provide the NUTRIENTS needed for good health. Nutritionists have devised the Food Guide Pyramid to help people achieve a balanced diet. By choosing a variety of foods from each of the pyramid's five food groups and by eating the right number of servings from each group, you can get enough of the nutrients your body needs. When planning what you will eat, consider variety and moderation as well as balance. Select different foods from the various food groups over time, and limit your intake of such nutrients as FATS, SODIUM, and added SUGARS. (See also DIETARY GUIDELINES.)

▶ BETA CAROTENE

RISK FACTORS
▶ ▶ ▶ ▶ ▶ ▶

HEALTHY CHOICES
■●●●●●●●●●●●

Beta carotene is a NUTRIENT, found in many vegetables and fruits, that the body converts to VITAMIN A. Once converted, it performs all the functions of vitamin A, which include promoting normal development of bones and teeth, maintaining healthy cell structure in the skin and mucous membranes, and aiding normal vision.

Beta carotene may have additional benefits as an antioxidant. An *antioxidant* is a substance that helps the body fight *free radicals,* unstable molecules that can damage cells. Free radicals form in the body during normal metabolism through exposure to various damaging external factors such as X rays, cigarette smoke, alcohol, and pollutants. The antioxidant activity of beta carotene may play a role in preventing cancer and heart disease; it may also help strengthen the immune system. Studies have found, however, that taking beta carotene as a supplement does not lower cancer risk and may even increase its risk in smokers. Therefore, doctors recommend eating foods that contain this nutrient as part of a BALANCED DIET.

Beta carotene is one of the PHYTOCHEMICALS found in vegetables and other plants. Good dietary sources of beta carotene are dark green, leafy vegetables such as kale, broccoli, and spinach, and dark yellow or orange fruits and vegetables such as carrots, sweet potatoes, winter squash, apricots, and cantaloupe. The National Cancer Institute and the U.S. Department of Agriculture recommend five ½-cup (118 ml) daily servings of such nutrient-rich fruits and vegetables, which would supply 5 to 6 grams of beta carotene. (See also VITAMINS.)

▶ BEVERAGES

Beverages, also called drinks, are consumed to meet the body's need for WATER and other NUTRIENTS. Nutrition experts recommend drinking at least eight glasses of water or other nonalcoholic, caffeine-free beverages a day, and more during periods of exercise or hot weather. An adequate beverage intake helps maintain good health and prevents DEHYDRATION, a condition in which the body's water level becomes dangerously low. The nutritional value of beverages varies, however (see illustration: Varied Nutritional Value of Beverages). Milk and fruit juice, for example, offer valuable nutrients, whereas soft drinks are very low in nutrients and can be high in CALORIES.

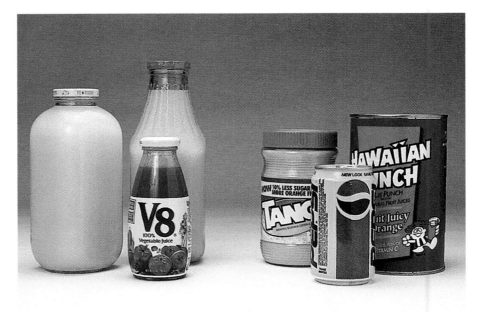

Varied Nutritional Value of Beverages. *Fruit and vegetable juices are much more nutritious than sodas and fruit-flavored drinks.*

HEALTHY CHOICES
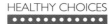

Water Water is essential to good health. While some people believe that bottled water is superior to or safer than tap water, studies have shown that this is not necessarily true. However, tap water may contain chemicals that are unhealthy or unpleasant-tasting. A filter can be used to remove these chemicals. The mineral content of any water is not nutritionally significant; however, the fluoride added to many community water supplies provides a health bonus by helping to prevent tooth decay. Some bottled waters have added carbonation (bubbles) or fruit flavorings.

Soft Drinks Soft drinks are America's most popular beverages, especially among people between the ages of 12 and 34. The average consumption is more than 16 ounces (about 475 ml) per person per day. Although many are sugar free and caffeine free, soft drinks are still the leading source of added SUGAR in the American diet. Regular soft drinks contain between 32 and 44 grams of sugar, so there are about 120 to 170 calories in each 12-ounce (355-ml) can. Diet soft drinks use ARTIFICIAL SWEETENERS such as saccharin or aspartame (NutraSweet®) in place of sugar. Soft drinks contain very few nutrients besides sugar, so they are often said to provide "empty" calories. Soft drinks are also the second leading source of the stimulant *caffeine.* Caffeine is a *diuretic,* a substance that removes fluid from the body; therefore, too much caffeine can lead to DEHYDRATION. Although a moderate intake of soft drinks should not pose health problems, nutritionists recommend that soft drinks not take the place of more nutritious beverages in the diet (especially milk for children and teenagers).

HEALTHY CHOICES
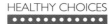

Fruit and Vegetable Drinks Fruit drinks and juices can be a healthy alternative to soft drinks, but their nutritional content varies greatly. Reading labels carefully to see what nutrients you are getting will help you select the most nutritious fruit drinks. Fresh or frozen fruit juices that are 100 percent juice are generally more nutritious than those labeled "fruit drink." A cup of orange juice, for example, provides 1.8 grams of protein, essential VITAMINS and MINERALS, and just 88 calories. A flavored fruit drink, on the other hand, may be only 10 percent natural fruit juices. Many people also enjoy vegetable juices, such as tomato and carrot juices.

HEALTHY CHOICES
●●●●●●●●●●●●

Milk Milk is a nutritious beverage. It is especially beneficial to children and teenagers (if they are not allergic to it) because it provides the calcium necessary for strong bones and teeth. A cup of milk provides about 300 milligrams of calcium, one-third of the amount needed each day for healthy bones. It also contains almost 9 grams of protein, assorted vitamins (including A, C, and D), iron, and 159 calories. A cup of skim milk, which has nearly all naturally occurring FATS removed, is a low-calorie alternative to whole milk, having 89 calories and all the essential vitamins and minerals, including calcium.

Tea and Coffee Tea and coffee, when consumed without cream, sugar, or other additives, have few or no calories and no significant food value. Although both beverages naturally contain caffeine, they are available in decaffeinated forms. Herbal teas, such as those made with peppermint and chamomile, contain no caffeine and are sometimes recommended for treating specific health problems or improving general health, and some people enjoy their flavors. No claims about the healing powers of herbs have been proven, however. (See also CAFFEINE, 7.)

▶ BODYBUILDING

Bodybuilding is a sport that uses certain types of STRENGTH TRAINING to increase muscle mass. The goal is a well-defined, highly muscled, and symmetrical body. This activity is becoming popular among both men and women.

The goal of bodybuilding differs from that of strength training. Strength training programs aim to develop muscle tone and STRENGTH, while bodybuilding has more to do with the aesthetics of muscle definition and form.

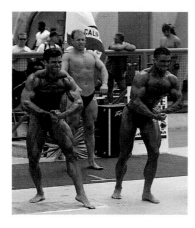

Bodybuilding Competition. *In professional competitions, judges evaluate bodybuilders' muscle definition, shape, and size as well as overall body proportions.*

RISK FACTORS
▶ ▶ ▶ ▶ ▶ ▶

The Regimen for Bodybuilding This sport requires intense, specialized techniques that use free weights or resistance machines. Hours of daily effort are necessary to achieve and maintain the desired muscle size and definition. Changing one's BODY COMPOSITION is an important part of bodybuilding: A very low proportion of body fat is considered desirable. Diet is consequently a crucial part of a bodybuilder's training program.

The Risks of Bodybuilding Like all sports that involve weights, bodybuilding does little to develop cardiovascular FITNESS. In addition, bodybuilders sometimes lose muscle and joint FLEXIBILITY as they add muscle mass. To promote total fitness, a bodybuilder's routine must include flexibility exercises and AEROBIC EXERCISES.

The use of *anabolic steroids* among bodybuilders is widespread. Many participants are tempted to take these potentially dangerous drugs because they help build muscle bulk. The possible side effects of anabolic steroids, including harmful physical and emotional changes, have led many bodybuilding organizations to ban their use. Participants may be required to take a drug test before a competition and will be disqualified if they have been taking steroids. In 1998 attention was focused on the DIETARY SUPPLEMENT *creatine*, which seems to allow athletes in training to build muscle mass at a higher-than-normal rate. Medical experts are cautious about recommending its use, since it has not undergone any rigorous testing. Possible harmful effects, especially on children and teenagers (who are still growing), are unknown. (See also ANAEROBIC EXERCISE; STEROIDS, 7.)

▶ BODY COMPOSITION

Body composition means the proportions of the major components of the body, especially the ratio of lean tissue to fat tissue. Body composition is usually expressed as the percentage of body weight that is fat.

Body Fat   The body needs a certain amount of fat for survival. It is essential for storing certain NUTRIENTS and converting them into energy, providing insulation for the body, and protecting internal organs. On the other hand, too much BODY FAT is unhealthy. Excess fat increases the risk of many diseases, including heart disease, cardiovascular disease, high blood pressure, diabetes, and certain cancers. The location of excess fat is also important: Fat around the abdomen represents a greater health risk than does fat elsewhere on the body.

RISK FACTORS
▶ ▶ ▶ ▶ ▶ ▶

Although too much body fat is a health concern, ideas about "ideal" body composition are also complicated by personal and cultural factors. Many teens feel uncomfortable about the appearance of their bodies because of normal physical changes that occur during adolescence. This discomfort may be worsened by social pressures. In America, fashion often decrees unrealistically low body-fat levels, especially for women. In reality, ideal body composition differs greatly from person to person (see illustration: Body Types). (See also EATING DISORDERS; PUBERTY, 6.)

Body Types. *Hereditary factors have a great deal to do with a person's body composition, which is also affected by diet and level of fitness. Three examples of the wide variety of body types are shown here: tall and thin (left), average height and muscular (center), and short and stocky (right).*

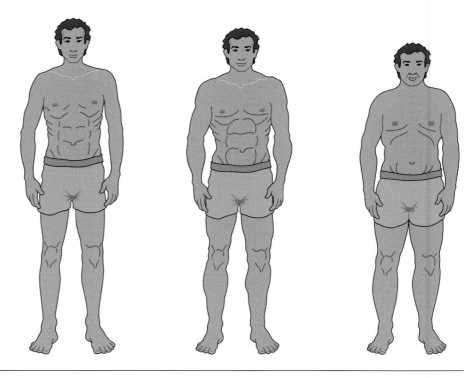

The appropriate proportion of body fat is one that is consistent with optimal health over a person's lifespan. In general, the acceptable range for men is between 10 and 18 percent of total weight; for women, it is between 18 and 25 percent. People at or above the top of these ranges are generally considered OVERWEIGHT for health purposes and should start a WEIGHT MANAGEMENT program that includes a healthy diet and regular, moderate physical activity. Exercise that develops cardiovascular FITNESS can help change body composition. With exercise, the percentage of fat tissue decreases while the percentage of lean tissue increases.

Measuring Body Composition   Techniques for measuring body composition include the *fatfold* (or skinfold) *test, hydrostatic* (or underwater) *weighing,* and *electric conductivity* (or bioelectrical impedance). The BODY MASS INDEX (BMI), the ratio of weight (in kilograms) divided by height (in meters) squared, is a common way to estimate healthy weight ranges. BMI does not, however, measure the proportion of fat to muscle tissue in the body. (See also DIETS; WEIGHT ASSESSMENT.)

▶ BODY FAT

RISK FACTORS
▶ ▶ ▶ ▶ ▶ ▶

When the body takes in more CALORIES from food than it needs to meet its energy needs, it converts the excess into body fat and stores it in *fat cells.* Over time, consuming more calories than the body needs causes the fat cells to increase in size, building up a layer of *adipose* (fatty) *tissue* around the body. Excessive body fat is associated with heart disease and several other health problems. Excess abdominal fat represents a more significant health risk than does fat in other parts of the body.

Formation of Body Fat   Energy can be produced for the body by three different substances: *amino acids,* which are also the building blocks of PROTEIN; GLUCOSE, the body's working CARBOHYDRATE; and *lipids,* which is the scientific name given to fats and closely related substances. Excess amounts of amino acids are not used to build and repair body cells. Instead, they are broken down and stored as body fat. Glucose, while it is the easiest energy source for the body to use, can be stored only in limited amounts as glycogen. Glycogen is saved in the liver and, to some extent, in the muscles themselves. Because fat cells are expandable, lipids can be stored in virtually unlimited amounts. Excess lipids, as well as amino acids and glucose from the diet, are often metabolized into storable lipids or body fat.

The fat cells of the body serve useful functions besides energy storage. They provide heat insulation under the skin and safety cushioning around the vital organs. Their major function, however, is to be the reserve storehouse for the body's energy needs; fat cells release lipids to provide physical energy when it is needed.

Lipids in the Body   There are different kinds of lipids, and they are important in many different ways. Lipids are a basic substance in all body cells and are necessary to help the body use some minerals and vitamins. Some lipids play a key part in producing hormones, which regulate certain body processes. An important part of lipids, called *fatty acids,* is used for energy storage and production. However, excessive amounts of fats in the blood can contribute to the development of atherosclerosis, heart attacks, and strokes. In addition, carrying too much body fat forces the heart to work harder to nourish the additional living tissue.

HEALTHY CHOICES
●●●●●●●●●●●●

Because of the various health problems associated with being overweight, medical experts recommend that only 10 to 18 percent of a man's weight should be in the form of body fat. For women, this number should be 18 to 25 percent. Various WEIGHT ASSESSMENT methods are used to determine how much of a person's weight comes from body fat. People who need to trim body fat can do so by burning more calories through physical activity and by consuming fewer calories in food. (See also BODY COMPOSITION; BODY MASS INDEX; CHOLESTEROL; ENERGY, FOOD; FATS; FATS, OILS, AND SWEETS; RISK FACTORS; ATHEROSCLEROSIS, 3; HEART DISEASE, 3.)

▶ BODY MASS INDEX

Body mass index (BMI) is the ratio of weight (in kilograms) divided by height (in meters) squared. BMI applies to both men and women 18 years of age and older. Health professionals use BMI to evaluate whether people are at risk for health problems associated with weight.

RISK FACTORS
▶ ▶ ▶ ▶ ▶ ▶

Assessing BMI is important because too much body weight increases the risk of heart disease, high blood pressure, diabetes, some cancers, and

BODY MASS INDEX CHART FOR ADULTS																	
BMI =	19	20	21	22	23	24	25	26	27	28	29	30	31	32	33	34	35
Weight (lbs.)																	
58	91	96	100	105	110	115	119	124	129	134	138	143	148	153	158	162	167
59	94	99	104	109	114	119	124	128	133	138	143	148	153	158	163	168	173
60	97	102	107	112	118	123	128	133	138	143	148	153	158	163	168	174	179
61	100	106	111	116	122	127	132	137	143	148	153	158	164	169	174	180	185
62	104	109	115	120	126	131	136	142	147	153	158	164	169	175	180	186	191
63	107	113	118	124	130	135	141	146	152	158	163	169	175	180	186	191	197
64	110	116	122	128	134	140	145	151	157	163	169	174	180	186	192	197	204
65	114	120	126	132	138	144	150	156	162	168	174	180	186	192	198	204	210
66	118	124	130	136	142	148	155	161	167	173	179	186	192	198	204	210	216
67	121	127	134	140	146	153	159	166	172	178	185	191	198	204	211	217	223
68	125	131	138	144	151	158	164	171	177	184	190	197	203	210	216	223	230
69	128	135	142	149	155	162	169	176	182	189	196	203	209	216	223	230	236
70	132	139	146	153	160	167	174	181	188	195	202	207	216	222	229	236	243
71	136	143	150	157	165	172	179	186	193	200	208	215	222	229	236	243	250
72	140	147	154	162	169	177	184	191	199	206	213	221	228	235	242	250	258
73	144	151	159	166	174	182	189	197	204	212	219	227	235	242	250	257	265
74	148	155	163	171	179	186	194	202	210	218	225	233	241	249	256	264	272
75	152	160	168	176	184	192	200	208	216	224	232	240	248	256	264	272	279
76	156	164	172	180	189	197	205	213	221	230	238	246	254	263	271	279	287

Height (in.)

other diseases. According to 1998 federal guidelines, a person with a BMI of 25 or less is considered at very low risk for health problems related to body weight (see chart: Body Mass Index Chart for Adults). A person with a BMI of 30 or above is considered at moderate to high risk. Health experts have developed a separate chart and way to use BMI to judge body weight for children and teens.

Use of Body Mass Index Data   Health professionals use BMI data to evaluate body weight. Weight problems represent a significant public health problem. In fact, by 1998 standards, about 55 percent of American adults—some 97 million people—are either overweight or obese.

Physicians use BMI data in combination with other information to assess health risks. For example, they evaluate a patient's RISK FACTORS, such as high blood cholesterol level and family history of certain health problems. They also consider the location of body fat: Excess abdominal fat represents a more significant health risk than does fat in other parts of the body. (See also WEIGHT ASSESSMENT.)

▶ BODY METABOLISM

Body metabolism includes all the biochemical changes that occur in the body to provide the energy needed for body processes. Metabolism consists of two processes: anabolism and catabolism. In *anabolism*, the simple products of DIGESTION are combined to form more complex substances. These substances are used by the body to grow, to repair body tissues, and to store energy. In *catabolism*, digested NUTRIENTS are further broken down to produce heat and energy. These processes are controlled by *hormones* and take place continuously.

Physical Activity and Metabolic Rate. *Exercise increases overall metabolic rate. A person who is in good physical shape burns calories at a faster rate than a person who rarely exercises.*

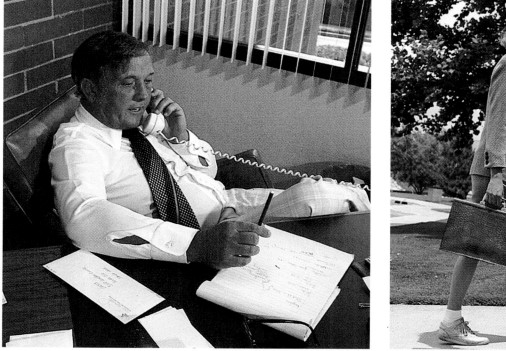

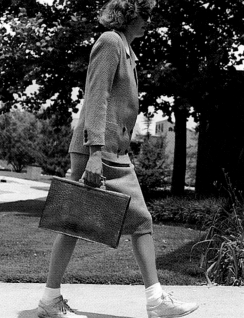

Measuring Metabolism   Basal metabolic rate is a measurement of the minimum amount of energy, counted in CALORIES, needed to maintain vital body processes, including circulation, breathing, and body temperature. It is measured while a person is at complete rest but not sleeping. The basal metabolic rate varies from person to person, depending on age, weight, genetics, and level of fitness. Men typically have higher rates than women.

The number of calories needed every day to support basal metabolism is surprisingly high: Approximately 50 to 70 percent of calories consumed are used to sustain the basic work of cells. The remaining calories are used for all voluntary activities, including exercise and sports. Any unused calories are stored as fat.

Factors Affecting Basal Metabolism   Many factors affect basal metabolic rate. Hormones secreted by the thyroid and adrenal glands have the most influence on the basal metabolic rate. An increase of hormones from either gland will raise body metabolism. For example, a surge of *adrenaline*, secreted by the adrenal glands in response to emotions such as anger or fear, will stimulate metabolism for a short period.

Both body temperature and environmental temperature also affect basal metabolic rate. A rise in body temperature of 1°F (0.56°C) increases basal metabolism about 7 percent, so a person with a fever will have increased energy needs. When the temperature of the air drops and a person does not put on extra clothes to slow the rate of heat loss, the body will increase its basal metabolic rate to produce more heat. Age also affects metabolic rate; it is higher in infancy and during puberty but then generally slows with age. Exercise temporarily raises the body's basal metabolic rate. Metabolism may be speeded up for as long as 24 hours after a prolonged period of physical activity.

Metabolism and Weight Management   Some researchers believe that people may have a given weight range, or *set point*, that is natural for their bodies. According to this theory, the body alters its basal metabolic rate to maintain weight at each person's particular set point. For example, if someone who has a high set point tries to lose weight by strict dieting, the body responds by burning calories more slowly and efficiently (thus slowing metabolism) to maintain a stable weight. This theory has not yet been proved. If it is true, it may help explain why dieting is so difficult for most individuals. The set-point theory does not mean, however, that losing weight is impossible. Increased physical activity is another important factor that raises the body's overall metabolic rate, including some increase in basal metabolic rate.

Metabolism and Fitness   All body tissues constantly undergo breakdown and repair; some have greater basal energy needs than others. The brain, major organs, and muscles require relatively larger amounts of energy in the form of calories. Bones and fat require less. A person who is in good shape usually has more muscle tissue and will, therefore, burn calories at a faster rate than someone who rarely exercises. Being fit thus contributes to a higher metabolic rate. Understanding this relationship may help people meet WEIGHT MANAGEMENT goals and plan sensible long-range

HEALTHY CHOICES

fitness programs. (See also AEROBIC EXERCISE; ENERGY, FOOD; ENERGY, PHYSICAL; EXERCISE; REST; METABOLISM, 1.)

▶ **BREAD, CEREAL, RICE, AND PASTA GROUP** The bread, cereal, rice, and pasta food group is one of the five major food groups in the FOOD GUIDE PYRAMID. It includes foods made from grains such as wheat, rice, oats, and corn. These foods are especially rich in complex CARBOHYDRATES, fairly rich in PROTEINS, and usually low in FATS and CALORIES. Many grain foods also contain significant amounts of VITAMINS, MINERALS, and FIBER.

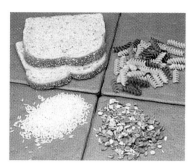

Bread, Cereal, Rice, and Pasta Group.

Nutrition from Bread, Cereal, Rice, and Pasta The bread, cereal, rice, and pasta group includes a number of different foods.

- *Breads* may be made from many grains, including wheat, corn, rye, and oats. *Yeast breads,* usually made from white and whole-wheat flours, are made with yeast. *Yeast* is a tiny plant that, when combined with other ingredients, causes bread to rise. *Quick breads,* such as muffins and corn bread, rise through the action of baking powder or other ingredients. *Flat breads,* including tortillas and pita bread, do not rise. White bread and many types of rolls are made from processed white processed flour. During processing, many important nutrients, especially B vitamins and IRON, are lost. Breads to which nutrients have been added are called *enriched breads. Whole-grain breads* are those in which unrefined grains have been used, so that important nutrients have not been lost. Whole-grain breads also contain *bran,* a part of the grain that provides both nutrients and fiber.

- *Cereals* are foods made from grains, usually eaten for breakfast. Some are ready sold to eat; others require cooking. As with white flour, the processing that many cereals go through destroys some of their nutrients. *Fortified cereals* are ones to which nutrients have been added. Choosing whole-grain and fortified cereals is the best way to ensure good nutrition from these foods.

- *Rice* is one so-called cereal grain. The outer coverings of *white rice,* the hull and the bran, have been removed. Because removing these coverings also removes many nutrients, most white rice is enriched with added vitamins. *Brown rice* has had the hull removed but retains the fiber-rich bran. This makes it more flavorful and more nutritious. It is important to use the proper amount of water when cooking rice to retain the rice's full nutritive value. Never rinse rice after you cook it, since rinsing can wash away important nutrients.

- *Pasta* is another member of the bread, cereal, rice, and pasta group. Spaghetti, macaroni, and noodles are all types of pasta. Many kinds are made from a type of wheat flour called semolina. Pasta dough can be cut into dozens of shapes and may be bought fresh or dried. Pasta may also be enriched with vitamins.

It should always be cooked according to the package directions, using the correct amount of water.

Daily Servings of Bread, Cereal, Rice, and Pasta The Food Guide Pyramid suggests making foods from the bread, cereal, rice, and pasta group the largest single part of your daily diet, recommending 6 to 11 servings for teenagers and young adults. A typical serving is 1 slice of bread; 1 ounce of dry cereal; or ½ cup of cooked cereal, rice, or pasta. The most healthful choices from this food group are usually the foods closest to their natural form. Whole grains are naturally low in fats and sugars, whereas highly processed grain foods are likely to have fat, sugar, or salt added to them. When you eat processed foods, check the labels to see how much fat and sugar they contain. For example, a doughnut is usually high in both, whereas a bagel contains little of either. Whole grains are also highest in fiber. It is a good idea to aim to get three of your daily servings of grains from whole-grain sources.

Although grain foods supply many important nutrients, they cannot make up a complete diet by themselves. Most grain foods contain some protein, but the proteins in grains are incomplete, lacking one or more of the essential *amino acids*. Therefore, foods from this group must be balanced with foods from the MEAT, POULTRY, FISH, DRY BEANS, EGGS, AND NUTS GROUP. Some grain foods are fortified with *folic acid,* a synthetic form of the nutrient *folate,* which is part of the VITAMIN B COMPLEX. (See also EXCHANGE SYSTEM; FATS, OILS, AND SWEETS; FRUIT GROUP; MILK, YOGURT, AND CHEESE GROUP; VEGETABLE GROUP; STARCH.)

▶ BREAKFAST

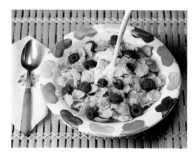

A Healthful Breakfast. *Many people enjoy cereal with fruit and milk in the morning. These are excellent breakfast choices, as are whole-grain breads and muffins, bagels, and fruit juices.*

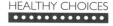
Breakfast is the day's first meal and one that nutritionists consider very important. Breakfast replenishes the blood's level of GLUCOSE, which the body's cells burn to produce energy.

Because 9 or more hours may have passed since the previous meal, breakfast provides the refueling the body needs to get through the morning. Glucose serves as the brain's principal source of energy. However, the brain does not store glucose. The food consumed at breakfast enables the body to produce a new supply of glucose that the brain can use to carry out mental activities. Replenishing the glucose supply also provides a source of energy for the muscles to carry out physical activities.

Breakfast Benefits Several research studies have highlighted the mental and physical benefits of breakfast. Eating breakfast has been associated with having a positive attitude toward work and being more productive in the late morning. People who eat breakfast tend to outperform those who don't at activities that require concentration, problem-solving abilities, or endurance. Children who eat breakfast on a regular basis tend to do better in school.

Breakfast has other benefits as well. Breakfast foods from the five food groups of the Food Guide Pyramid (such as cereal, milk, and fruit) contribute to a BALANCED DIET. People who skip breakfast when trying to lose weight may achieve the opposite effect. Several studies have shown that people who skip breakfast tend to snack and eat more high-CALORIE foods later in the day.

▶ BREAST MILK

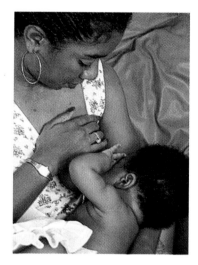

Breast-Feeding.

Breast milk is milk that is produced in a woman's *mammary glands* after she has given birth. Breast milk is the most complete food for babies. It is easy for infants to digest and provides virtually all the NUTRIENTS a baby needs as well as *antibodies* that protect the child from diseases. Breast milk also stimulates the development of the infant's gastrointestinal tract.

Breast milk provides about 600 CALORIES of food energy per day. It combines CARBOHYDRATES, FATS, and PROTEIN in a form that promotes an infant's proper growth and development. Breast milk also provides nearly all the VITAMINS, MINERALS, and WATER that an infant needs. Pediatricians generally recommend supplements of VITAMIN D, fluoride, and IRON.

A new mother usually does not produce milk until the third day after her child's birth. Until then, the breasts produce *colostrum,* a fatty substance containing white blood cells and antibodies from the mother's bloodstream that help protect the infant against bacterial infections and such viruses as colds.

Many pediatricians and family physicians recommend breast-feeding. In addition to providing valuable antibodies and essential nutrients, breast-feeding involves a physical closeness that strengthens the bond between mother and child. Breast-feeding can also improve the health of the mother, helping her recover more quickly from childbirth and lowering her risk of certain cancers. However, it is not recommended for a mother who is taking certain medications, who is addicted to alcohol or other drugs, or who has certain communicable diseases, such as tuberculosis or hepatitis. (See also ANTIBODY, **2**; BREAST-FEEDING, **6**.)

▶ BULIMIA

see EATING DISORDERS

▶ CALCIUM

Calcium is the most plentiful MINERAL in the human body. It plays an important role in a number of bodily functions, including blood clotting, muscle contraction, the transmission of nerve impulses, and the growth and maintenance of bones and teeth. About 99 percent of the calcium in the body is contained in the bones in the form of *calcium phosphate.* The remainder is found in the blood and other body fluids. The amount of calcium in the body is controlled by the actions of certain *hormones* and VITAMIN D. When the level of calcium in the blood is too low, the blood absorbs more from the intestines or bones.

Calcium in the Diet The recommended *adequate intake* for calcium is 500 to 800 mg per day for children under 9, 1300 mg per day for youths

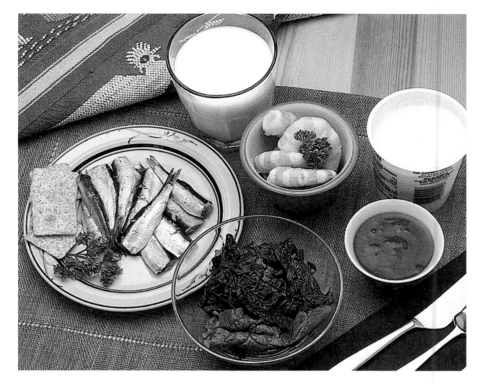

Sampling of Foods Rich in Calcium. *The recommended adequate intake for adults is 1,000 mg for people 19 to 50 years old and 1,200 mg after the age of 50. Foods rich in this mineral include sardines with bones, nonfat milk or yogurt, shrimp, and spinach.*

RISK FACTORS
► ► ► ► ► ►

HEALTHY CHOICES
■ ● ● ● ● ● ● ● ● ● ■ ●

from age 9 to 18, and 1000 mg per day for adults from age 19 to 50. After age 50, adults should get 1200 mg of calcium per day. An inadequate amount of calcium in the diet can result in bone degeneration and crippling deformities. Children and adolescents whose diets are extremely deficient in calcium may develop *rickets,* a condition that causes softening of the bones and bowing of the legs. Calcium deficiency this severe is rarely seen in the United States. A more common problem is *osteoporosis,* a condition found mostly in older adults, in which the bones lose calcium and become brittle and porous. Although almost everyone suffers some loss of bone mass after age 35, osteoporosis is most commonly diagnosed in women several years after *menopause.* Building strong bones by getting enough calcium during childhood and adolescence can help prevent osteoporosis later in life.

Most experts advise that men and women continue to eat calcium-rich foods throughout their lives in order to maintain adequate stores of calcium in the body. Calcium-rich foods include milk and other products from the MILK, YOGURT, AND CHEESE GROUP; green vegetables such as broccoli, spinach, and collard greens; and fish with edible bones, such as salmon and sardines. For example, an 8-ounce glass of milk contains about one-third of the calcium your body needs daily. A cup of cooked broccoli supplies about one-sixth of your daily calcium needs. Some other foods that are high in calcium are tofu, dry beans, and calcium-fortified juices.

Certain factors affect the body's ability to absorb calcium. Increased levels of vitamin D and phosphorus in the diet will aid the absorption of calcium. Too much protein and sodium in the diet can limit absorption. (See also RECOMMENDED DIETARY ALLOWANCE; VITAMINS; OSTEOPOROSIS, **3.**)

CALORIE

The calorie is a unit of heat energy. It is used to measure both stored energy (as in food) and energy expended (as by any living organism). In relation to nutrition, *calorie* generally refers to a unit of energy that is, technically speaking, a kilocalorie: the amount of heat needed to raise the temperature of 1 kilogram of water 1°C.

Calories are an important concept to understand in relation to diet. Your body needs enough of them in the form of food to provide adequate fuel for all of its energy expenditures. When you consume too many calories over a period of time, your body stores the excess, primarily in the form of BODY FAT, causing you to gain weight. When you burn more calories than you consume, you lose weight because fat cells are reduced in size as their fat is consumed to provide energy.

A constant body weight results from a long-term balance of calories consumed (energy intake) and calories burned (energy expenditure), a concept called the *energy balance equation*. The average adult burns between 1,500 and 3,000 calories a day. This number varies according to a wide range of factors, including age, sex, weight, activity level, and rate of BODY METABOLISM.

Calories and Energy Intake The energy values of specific foods are measured by determining how many calories they contain. This is done in a laboratory with a device called a *bomb calorimeter* in which small quantities of foods are burned. The heat they generate is then measured in calories.

Using this method, nutritionists have counted the calories contained in every imaginable kind of food. A teaspoon of sugar, for example, has 16 calories; a cup of 2 percent milk has 130; and a 3-ounce (85-g) hamburger patty has 245. Calorie counts such as these are available in diet and nutrition books, in many cookbooks, and on many food packages. They can be used to determine how many calories you consume daily.

Calories and Energy Expenditure In similar ways, researchers have calculated how many calories are burned in the course of specific activities. Basically, the more a body has to work, the more fuel it requires in the form of calories. The level of physical activity, or EXERCISE, is therefore one of the largest variables in a person's daily energy expenditure. The number of calories used during exercise depends on the intensity of the activity and on how frequently and for how long it is done.

Every physical activity burns calories at its own rate. For example, a 150-pound (68-kg) person burns roughly 240 calories an hour walking slowly (2 miles per hour), 440 calories an hour racewalking (4.5 miles per hour), 750 calories an hour jumping rope, and 920 calories an hour running (at 7 miles or 11 km per hour). The more strenuous the activity, the more calories it requires. However, even regular daily activities that are not usually thought of as exercise burn some calories: about 70 calories per hour watching television, 150 calories per hour doing homework, and 300 per hour doing heavy cleaning.

Balancing Intake and Expenditure Understanding the calorie values of foods and of exercise and other activities is critical to anyone concerned with WEIGHT MANAGEMENT. The essential fact is that every 3,500 calories you consume in excess of what you expend is converted to 1 pound of body fat. Therefore, to lose 10 pounds (4.5 kg), you would have to burn 35,000 (3,500 × 10) calories more than you consume over a period of time.

Although that figure seems high, even minor adjustments to eating and exercise can produce large shifts in the energy balance equation. For example, reducing calorie consumption by just 100 calories a day while engaging in just 3 hours of moderate exercise a week can produce a weight loss of 20 to 30 pounds in a year. Regular daily activities, such as walking to school, can be part of calorie-burning exercise. (See also DIETS; ENERGY, FOOD; ENERGY, PHYSICAL; WEIGHT-GAIN STRATEGY; WEIGHT-LOSS STRATEGY; METABOLISM, 1.)

► CARBOHYDRATES

Carbohydrates are one of the three main groups of *macronutrients,* nutrients that the body needs in large amounts. They are compounds of carbon, hydrogen, and oxygen atoms that are formed in quantity within all plants. Therefore, they are found in most foods from plant sources, although some animal-based foods, such as milk, also contain some carbohydrates. People have limited capacity to store carbohydrates; what cannot be used or held in the liver or the muscles tends to be turned into BODY FAT.

Carbohydrates perform four main functions, three of which are connected with energy. They are the most important source of energy for all body functions; they are necessary to allow efficient use of FATS as an energy source; and they protect PROTEINS from being used for energy in emergencies. Finally, in the form of fiber, they provide bulk needed to aid digestion.

Simple Carbohydrates Depending on their chemical structures, carbohydrates are either complex or simple. Simple carbohydrates are SUGARS, with as few as 6 carbon atoms per molecule. They are present in dairy products and in many foods from plant sources, especially fruits and certain root vegetables. Sugary foods also include foods made with added sugar, such as candy and soft drinks. These foods are often very high in CALORIES in relation to the nutrients they provide. Sugars are easy to digest and to convert to energy, but many sugary foods are low in other NUTRIENTS. Naturally sweet foods, such as fruit, usually have plenty of other nutrients in proportion to the number of calories they supply.

Complex Carbohydrates Complex carbohydrates are large molecules with many carbon atoms: The most complex of all, STARCHES, have about 200,000 per molecule. Starches are made up of many simple sugars linked together. They break down into sugars when they are digested. Foods rich in starch molecules include those found in the BREAD, CEREAL, RICE, AND PASTA GROUP as well as in the VEGETABLE GROUP. They usually contain many other valuable nutrients as well, including VITAMINS, MINERALS, and proteins. Many also contain water and fiber.

Like starch, FIBER is a complex carbohydrate found in most foods of plant origin. Unlike starch, however, fiber cannot be absorbed and used for energy because it is not broken down during digestion. Instead, it provides roughage that binds with solid wastes and aids in their elimination from the body.

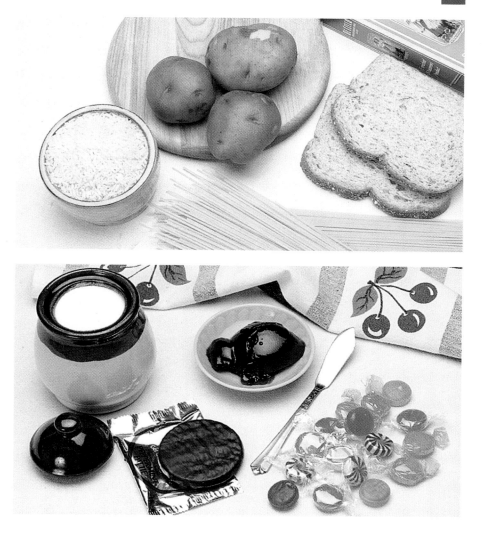

Complex and Simple Carbo-hydrates. *Complex carbohydrates are found in bread, rice, potatoes, and pasta. These foods have more nutritional value than the simple-carbohydrate foods made with refined sugar.*

HEALTHY CHOICES
● ● ● ● ● ● ● ● ● ● ●

Carbohydrates in the Diet Most nutritionists recommend that 55 to 60 percent of your total daily calories come from carbohydrates. Added sugars, however, should be consumed in moderation. Sugary foods such as candy bars do not provide many nutrients besides carbohydrates. You should choose foods high in complex carbohydrates or natural sugars to provide you with energy. People with diabetes, whose bodies have diffi-culty regulating the amount of sugar in their blood, must carefully man-age their intake of carbohydrates.

A diet high in complex carbohydrates can be both satisfying and nu-tritionally beneficial for athletes. Athletes often find it helpful to eat a diet extra high in carbohydrates—around 70 percent of total calories—for several days before an endurance athletic event. This has proved to be a reliable way to create energy reserves in muscles and thus extend the time that the body is able to maintain strenuous activity. Called *carbohydrate loading*, this practice is not recommended for teenage athletes.

RISK FACTORS
▶ ▶ ▶ ▶ ▶ ▶

Carbohydrates play an indirect role in tooth decay. Sugars and other carbohydrates can adhere to teeth and gums, providing a good environ-ment for bacteria to produce acids that can damage teeth. It is a good idea to brush your teeth after eating carbohydrate-rich foods. (See also ENERGY, FOOD; DENTAL PROBLEMS, 3; DIABETES, 3.)

··

▶ **CEREALS**   see BREAD, CEREAL, RICE, AND PASTA GROUP

··

▶ **CHOLESTEROL**   Cholesterol is a waxlike, fat-related substance that is an important part of all animal cells. Among its many roles, cholesterol helps the body produce *bile*, which aids in digestion. Cholesterol is also involved in creating certain *hormones*, VITAMIN D, and the outer coverings that protect nerve fibers. Although most of the cholesterol in your body is manufactured by your liver, cholesterol is also present in foods of animal origin, such as butter, eggs, meats, and cheeses. Foods that come from plants do not contain cholesterol.

RISK FACTORS
▶ ▶ ▶ ▶ ▶ ▶

Cholesterol in the Blood   Although cholesterol is essential to life, when too much of it circulates in the blood, it can create a fatty buildup, or plaque, on the inner walls of the arteries. This condition, known as *atherosclerosis,* can lead to stroke, coronary artery disease, or heart attack. (See also ATHEROSCLEROSIS, **3**; HEART DISEASE, **3**.)

Cholesterol is carried through the bloodstream by special molecules called *lipoproteins*. Two major types of lipoproteins are important cholesterol carriers. They are differentiated by their size and density. The larger is *low-density lipoprotein,* or LDL. It is associated with increased risk of atherosclerosis. For this reason, the cholesterol that LDL carries is referred to as "bad" cholesterol. Smaller and denser, *high-density lipoprotein,* or HDL, appears to carry excess cholesterol away from the artery walls and back to the liver, where it is processed and excreted. Because HDL performs a kind of cleanup function, its cholesterol is referred to as "good" cholesterol.

Cholesterol Levels   There are two types of blood tests that measure cholesterol levels. The simpler (and less expensive) test measures the total amount of cholesterol present in the blood. Fewer than 200 milligrams per deciliter (mg/dl) is usually considered healthy, while 240 mg/dl or more is considered a high cholesterol level. This test, however, makes no distinction between good and bad cholesterol.

The second test provides a "cholesterol profile," measuring how much cholesterol is carried by LDLs and how much by HDLs. This yields a "cholesterol ratio," for example, 130/30 or 4.3. Doctors usually consider the results of both tests before they decide on any treatment: A high HDL measure (which causes a low ratio) is a good sign and makes a high figure on the first test less worrisome.

RISK FACTORS
▶ ▶ ▶ ▶ ▶ ▶

Controlling Cholesterol Problems   A variety of factors can influence levels of cholesterol in the blood. An important factor is diet, but others, such as heredity (the cholesterol level typical of your family); diseases such as *diabetes* and *hypothyroidism,* exercise level; and excess weight are also known to influence cholesterol. While the effects of heredity and disease cannot easily be changed, doctors can help people control their cholesterol level by recommending exercise, weight loss, and, above all, dietary change.

HEALTHY CHOICES
■ ● ● ● ● ● ● ● ● ● ■

Exercise and weight loss have both been shown to help elevate the level of "good" (HDL) cholesterol in the bloodstream. By contrast, dietary

SATURATED FAT AND CHOLESTEROL CONTENTS OF FOODS

Food	Saturated Fat (g)	Cholesterol (mg)
Cheddar cheese (1 oz)	6	29
Mozzarella, part skim (1 oz)	3	16
Whole milk (1 cup)	5	33
Skim milk (1 cup)	Trace	4
Egg, 1	2	213
Butter (1 tbsp)	7	31
Mayonnaise (1 tbsp)	2	7
Tuna in oil (3 oz)	1	25
Tuna in water (3 oz)	Trace	25
Lean ground beef, broiled (3 oz)	6	73
Chicken, roasted, no skin (3 oz)	2	75
Beef liver, braised (3 oz)	2	331

Source: Adapted from Roberta Larson Duyff. 1998. *The American Dietetic Association's Complete Food and Nutrition Guide.* Minneapolis, MN: Chronimed.

HEALTHY CHOICES

HEALTHY CHOICES

HEALTHY CHOICES

CONSULT A PHYSICIAN

change focuses mostly on reducing LDL cholesterol. The most effective single step is to reduce the intake of *saturated fats,* which cause the liver to produce more LDL cholesterol. Cholesterol-rich foods should also be avoided, though the evidence is that saturated FATS are the greater contributor to blood cholesterol. The DIETARY GUIDELINES for Americans suggest that fats should account for no more than 30 percent of calories consumed, with 10 percent or less of daily calories coming from saturated fat, and that daily cholesterol intake should not exceed 300 milligrams (see chart: Saturated Fat and Cholesterol Contents of Foods).

While saturated fat tends to raise levels of LDL cholesterol, *monounsaturated fats* (such as those found in olive and canola oils) can actually lower it. Other foods that can reduce your level of LDL cholesterol are those high in soluble FIBER (such as oatmeal and oat bran) and foods that contain soy protein (such as tofu). For people who cannot lower their blood cholesterol to a healthy level through changes in diet and lifestyle, doctors may prescribe drugs that reduce LDL cholesterol. (See also BODY FAT; FAST FOOD; FOOD LABELING; MEAT, POULTRY, FISH, DRY BEANS, EGGS, AND NUTS GROUP; RISK FACTORS.)

▶ **CROSS TRAINING** Cross training is working out regularly at more than one athletic activity. This method of training has several advantages. It provides good overall conditioning by exercising more muscle groups; it reduces the risk of injury; and it helps alleviate the boredom that can occur with a single-activity program. RUNNING and SWIMMING are examples of well-matched cross-training activities. Running builds lower-body STRENGTH and *muscular endurance,* while swimming conditions the upper body. Both activities help develop cardiovascular ENDURANCE.

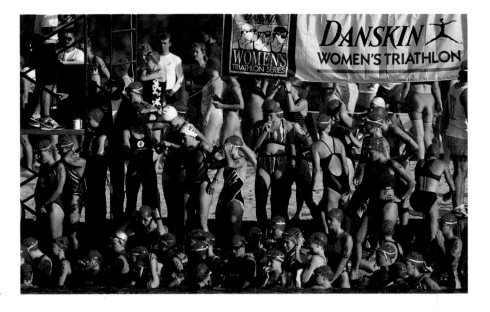

Triathlons. *Triathlons—swimming 2 miles, cycling 100 miles, and running a 26-mile marathon—are cross-training competitions that include some of the most physically fit athletes in the world.*

HEALTHY CHOICES
●○●○●○●○●○●○●○

When planning a cross-training schedule, choose activities that work different parts of the body. Continually performing one activity can put too much stress on the same muscles and joints, thus increasing the risk of injury. By alternating rowing with CYCLING every other day, for instance, you would give the different muscle groups a rest between workouts. Also, if an injury occurs at one activity, it may be possible to continue to maintain fitness by engaging in the alternate activity while healing. (See also AEROBIC EXERCISE; EXERCISE; FITNESS; FITNESS TRAINING; SPORTS AND FITNESS; STRENGTH TRAINING.)

▶ CYCLING

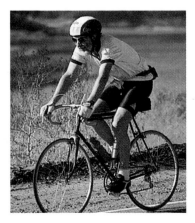

Cycling. *Cycling can be a very pleasant way to strengthen the heart and lungs and exercise leg muscles.*

Cycling, or bicycle riding, is an excellent form of AEROBIC EXERCISE. It strengthens the heart and lungs, builds leg muscles, and burns about 400 calories per hour. Nearly anyone in good health can ride a bicycle. Cycling, however, requires more expensive equipment than some other aerobic activities, and it is not suitable for all weather conditions. Many fitness cyclists use indoor stationary bikes to avoid bad weather and road hazards.

Preparing to Ride Cycling includes casual riding, racing, and mountain biking (riding over rough, hilly terrain) as well as riding for fitness. For fitness cycling, choose a bike that has 10 to 12 speeds. A good-quality bicycle can cost several hundred dollars, so make sure that the one you choose fits your needs.

When you begin a cycling program, ride on paved roads over flat or gently rolling terrain. Start out riding for 30 to 45 minutes (less if you have not been exercising) three times a week, and work up slowly to an hour or more. Pedal in a gear that allows a pace of about 60 to 80 pedal revolutions per minute. Pedaling too fast or too hard can lead to muscle soreness; pedaling in a very high gear can also cause "biker's knee," a pain around the kneecap. (See also SPORTS INJURIES.)

Cycling Safety   Safety is an important concern for cyclists. Each year, more than 750 Americans are killed in cycling accidents. About 65,000 people are taken to emergency rooms, and 7,700 are admitted to hospitals, annually because of head injuries related to cycling. While riding, always wear a safety helmet approved by the American National Standards Institute (ANSI). In addition, wear brightly colored clothing, keep an eye on traffic, and always use hand signals. Be alert to hazardous road conditions such as potholes, ice, storm drains, and railroad tracks. (See also FITNESS; FITNESS TRAINING; HEART RATE.)

▶ **DAIRY PRODUCTS**   see MILK, YOGURT, AND CHEESE GROUP

▶ **DEHYDRATION**   Dehydration is a condition in which the percentage of water in a person's body is dangerously low. WATER is essential to good health and should account for between 55 and 75 percent of an adult's weight. A reduction of even 2 percent of the body's water content can reduce the ability of cells and tissues to function properly. Severe dehydration can cause death.

Causes and Symptoms   Dehydration can be caused by excessive perspiration during exercise. The amount of water lost through perspiration is likely to be higher in hot or humid weather, but it is possible to become dehydrated this way even in cold weather. Large amounts of water can also be lost when a person experiences persistent *vomiting* or *diarrhea*.

Symptoms of dehydration include severe thirst, dry lips and tongue, increased heart rate and breathing rate, low blood pressure, dizziness, nausea, and confusion. A frequent complication of dehydration is the loss of salt and other vital substances in the body, causing lethargy, headache, cramps, and pallor.

Fluid Replacement Prevents Dehydration. *Adequate fluid intake during exercise is very important. Without enough fluids, the body can become dehydrated, a condition that results in fatigue and reduced athletic ability.*

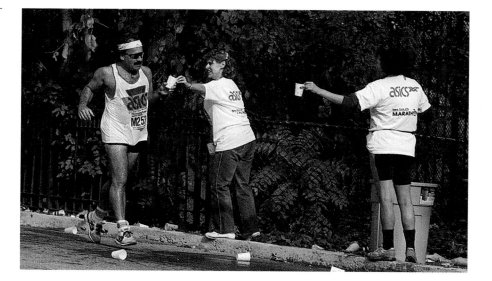

Prevention   The sense of thirst normally indicates when the water content of the body is low. When water loss is rapid, however, the normal thirst mechanism may not keep up with water loss and may fail to warn of dehydration. The best way to prevent dehydration, therefore, is to drink water before, during, and after exercise, especially in hot weather. Check your weight before and after a workout. A sensible guideline is to drink a pint (about 0.5 L) of water for each pound (about 0.5 kg) lost during exercise. Sports beverages can also be effective for preventing and treating dehydration. (See also BEVERAGES; EXERCISE AND HEAT INJURY.)

▶ DIET AIDS

Diet aids, which include prescription and over-the-counter pills, powders, supplements, and surgical procedures, are tried by a large number of OVERWEIGHT people in search of a fast and easy way to lose weight. Although some are effective to a certain degree, many are not, and all have drawbacks that must be carefully weighed against their possible benefits. In some cases, the disadvantages of diet aids are serious enough to justify their use only by very obese people. Because of these risks, diet aids should be used only under the guidance of a physician. For any diet aid to work, it must be part of a weight-loss plan that includes a reduced CALORIE intake and increased EXERCISE.

Among the drugs used for weight loss are over-the-counter *diet pills* intended to act as *appetite suppressants;* that is, they block a person's desire to eat. The Food and Drug Administration has found that appetite suppressants containing the decongestant phenylpropanolamine are safe and somewhat effective diet aids. In some people, however, this drug may cause a dangerous rise in blood pressure. Two other appetite suppressants, fenfluramine (Pondimin) and dexfenfluramine (Redux), were recently removed from the market after they were linked with potentially deadly heart valve disorders.

Appetite suppressants containing synthetic drugs called *amphetamines* are best used under medical supervision and with extreme caution. Amphetamines are strongly addictive *stimulants* that can have unpleasant side effects, such as sleeplessness, irritability, and depression. In addition, without changes in LIFESTYLE, most people gain back the weight they lose by using amphetamines.

Some people use an herbal supplement known as *ephedrine,* or ma huang, as an appetite suppressant. This herb works much as amphetamines do but can be purchased without a prescription. High doses of ephedrine, however, can cause dangerous heart and nervous system problems, including heart attacks, seizures, and stroke. (See also METHAMPHETAMINES, 7.)

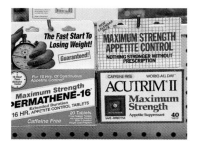

Appetite Suppressants. *There are many appetite suppressants on the market, but they are rarely good choices for long-term weight loss and overall good health. They should be used only with a physician's guidance.*

Diuretics and laxatives are sometimes used as diet aids, particularly by people who suffer from an EATING DISORDER called *bulimia.* Using these drugs is not an effective way to lose weight that consists of excess BODY FAT. Instead, they promote the loss of water weight and can cause DEHYDRATION. Both can be harmful if taken for any length of time. The thyroid hormone *thyroxine* is sometimes prescribed by physicians to help people whose excess weight is caused by an underactive thyroid gland. Very few people, however, are overweight due to poor thyroid function. (See also THYROID DISORDERS, 3; DIURETIC, 7; LAXATIVES, 7.)

Other diet aids include vitamin-enriched candies (sold as appetite suppressants), products high in FIBER (intended to make the stomach feel full), and various powders that are mixed with milk and consumed in place of meals. Several manufacturers produce lines of DIET FOODS that can help reduce weight by providing controlled portions of low-calorie foods. These types of foods are expensive; equivalent or superior low-calorie meals are easy to make at home.

Surgical procedures to help people lose weight include *liposuction* (suctioning fat deposits from under the skin), wiring the jaw closed, stapling the stomach to make it smaller, bypassing part of the intestine to limit the process of DIGESTION, and inserting a balloon in the stomach to make it feel full. These procedures all involve some risk and can produce complications. They are meant to be undertaken as a last resort by extremely overweight people.

Investigate any diet aid carefully before trying it. Most are ineffective in the long run, and some are dangerous. There is no magic pill or quick-fix procedure that can substitute for eating a well-balanced, low-calorie diet and engaging in regular exercise. (See also APPETITE; DIETARY GUIDELINES; DIETS; FAD DIETS; NUTRITION; WEIGHT-LOSS STRATEGY; WEIGHT MANAGEMENT.)

▶ DIETARY GUIDELINES

Dietary guidelines are recommendations designed to encourage healthy eating habits. Issued by government or scientific agencies to promote good health through proper NUTRITION, dietary guidelines can help people control their weight and reduce the occurrence of certain diseases.

Dietary guidelines cover the types and quantities of food that should be eaten daily. Often, they suggest how each day's calories should be distributed among the categories of NUTRIENTS: FATS, PROTEINS, CARBOHYDRATES, VITAMINS, and MINERALS. They may recommend limiting the consumption of foods such as fats, SALT, and SUGAR, that are known to contribute to certain diseases. They may also emphasize certain foods that are essential to maintaining good health, such as those high in FIBER.

The nature of dietary guidelines has changed over the years. In the 1940s, government authorities were concerned primarily about inadequate nutrition in the population. Today, they are also concerned about excessive consumption of certain foods. Guidelines issued by different organizations may vary, depending upon the health concerns they address.

The *Dietary Guidelines for Americans*, produced by the U.S. Department of Agriculture (USDA) and the U.S. Department of Health and Human Services, encourage people to eat a balanced diet and to limit their consumption of less nutritious foods. The official guidelines as of 1995 are summarized as follows:

HEALTHY CHOICES

> *Eat a variety of foods.* You can use the FOOD GUIDE PYRAMID to help you choose the best amounts of different kinds of foods.
> *Balance the food you eat with physical activity. Maintain or improve your weight.* Thirty minutes or more of moderate EXERCISE, most days of the week, contributes greatly to overall health.
> *Choose a diet with plenty of grain products, vegetables, and fruits.* These foods, which are high in many vital nutrients, should supply most of your daily CALORIES.

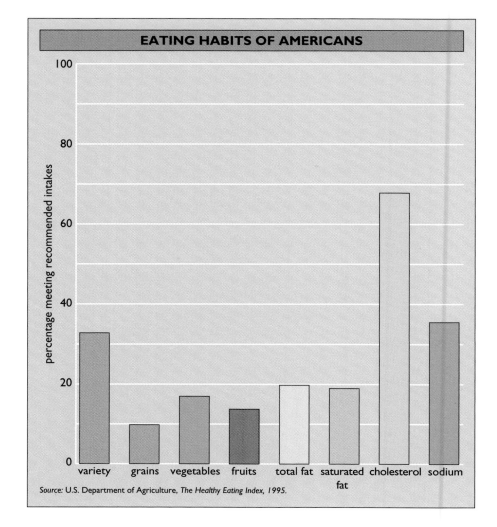

EATING HABITS OF AMERICANS

Source: U.S. Department of Agriculture, *The Healthy Eating Index*, 1995.

▶ *Choose a diet low in fat, saturated fat, and cholesterol.* Diets high in fats and CHOLESTEROL are associated with heart disease.

▶ *Choose a diet moderate in sugars.* This advice is especially important for people whose daily calorie needs are low.

▶ *Choose a diet moderate in salt and sodium.* High salt intake can contribute to high blood pressure in some people.

▶ *If you drink alcoholic beverages, do so in moderation.* Some people, such as children and adolescents, problem drinkers, and pregnant women, should not drink alcohol at all. (See also AL-COHOL, 7.)

The full text of *Dietary Guidelines for Americans* provides information on why each of the guidelines is important and how to follow them. The Healthy Eating Index, published by the USDA in 1995, compared Americans' actual eating habits to the diet recommended in the *Dietary Guidelines for Americans*. The graph on this page shows what percentage of the people studied met the guidelines' recommended intakes in selected areas (see graph: Eating Habits of Americans). (See also RECOMMENDED DIETARY ALLOWANCE; WEIGHT MANAGEMENT.)

▶ DIETARY SUPPLEMENTS

Dietary supplements are products that people take in addition to the foods they eat in order to gain some health benefit. These supplements may or may not be recommended by a physician. Supplements include VITAMINS, MINERALS, herbs, enzymes, or amino acids. Dietary supplements—which must, by law, be clearly labeled as such—are sold as pills, tablets, capsules, liquids, and powders.

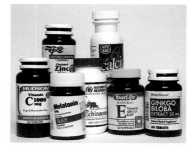

Dietary Supplements. *Although many dietary supplements are available and some can be helpful, the best way to get the vitamins you need is through a varied, balanced diet.*

Kinds of Supplements Vitamins and minerals are the most widely used dietary supplements. Physicians may advise some people to take a daily supplement. Usually, a doctor advises a supplement that provides no more than 100 percent of the RECOMMENDED DIETARY ALLOWANCES (RDA) for various nutrients. RDAs are the nutrient amounts recommended daily for healthy people. Women over age 50 may be advised to take calcium supplements to help prevent bone loss, which may lead to osteoporosis. Pregnant women, too, may take calcium supplements as well as iron and *folic acid* supplements.

Other dietary supplements include such herbs as echinacea, ginkgo biloba, and *melatonin,* a synthetic form of a human hormone. Scientific evidence about the effectiveness and safe dosage of herbal supplements is limited. Some herbal supplements may have harmful side effects.

Use and Abuse of Dietary Supplements Americans spend billions of dollars each year on dietary supplements. Many people take supplements as "insurance" to protect against dietary deficiencies. Others take specific supplements on a physician's recommendation. Still others take these products in hopes of preventing diseases such as cancer.

While dietary supplements can help people meet nutritional goals, they cannot serve as an adequate substitute for a BALANCED DIET or skilled medical care. Moreover, some people take excessive quantities of supplements, well beyond the recommended dosage. Overdoses of some supplements can damage the body or even cause death.

Regulation of Dietary Supplements Supplements are not regulated by the Food and Drug Administration (FDA) in the same way that drugs are. Dietary supplements need not be registered with or approved by the FDA before they can be sold. However, the law does require that manufacturers be truthful in their label information. (See also OSTEOPOROSIS, **3.**)

▶ DIET FOOD

Diet food is intended primarily for weight loss. Many food manufacturers produce specially prepared diet foods that are low in CALORIES and FATS and/or come in closely controlled portions. For this reason, diet foods are often called *low-fat foods* or *low-calorie foods.*

Diet Food Labels Federal regulations have helped to standardize food labels and make them more accurate and less misleading. Nevertheless, manufacturers' terminology can still be confusing, and it is important to read labels carefully in order to make informed choices about the variety of diet foods available.

By law, any food labeled "low-calorie" must have no more than 40 calories per serving. A food labeled "reduced-calorie" must have at least

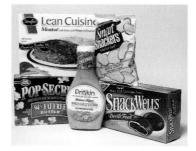

Diet Food. *A variety of foods is now available to meet the needs of people on weight-loss diets.*

25 percent fewer calories than the food to which it is being compared. "Low-fat" foods must contain no more than 3 grams of fat per serving.

A food labeled "light" (or "lite") may have one-third fewer calories or half as much fat as the food to which it is being compared. However, if at least half the calories of the regular version of the food come from fat, the reduction in the light version must be at least 50 percent of the fat content. "Light" may also mean that the sodium content of a low-calorie, low-fat food has been reduced by half.

Prepared Diet Foods Prepared diet foods come in many different forms. A variety of diet frozen entrees is available. Diet foods such as soda, candy, and yogurt are often made with an ARTIFICIAL SWEETENER. Diet snack foods are those that have been baked (not fried) to reduce the amount of fats. Many diet desserts are on the market, including those in which skim milk has been used in place of whole milk or those made with fat substitutes.

Since 1996, a synthetic fat called *olestra* has aroused considerable interest and controversy. Olestra is different from all other approved fat substitutes currently on the market. It offers the flavor and cooking characteristics of real fats and oils but has no calories. However, critics of olestra note that it is indigestible and may interfere with the body's absorption of certain nutrients. So far, the Food and Drug Administration has approved olestra for use only in snack foods.

Diet Food Use Diet foods should be used only as part of a WEIGHT-LOSS STRATEGY that includes a well-balanced diet and regular EXERCISE. FAD DIETS, popular diets that do not provide complete NUTRITION, can be dangerous. (See also APPETITE; DIET AIDS; DIETARY GUIDELINES; DIETS; FOOD LABELING; OVERWEIGHT; WEIGHT MANAGEMENT.)

▶ DIETS

A diet is the combination of all the foods an individual eats on a regular basis. A healthful and balanced eating plan is essential to maintaining good health, repairing damaged body tissues, and satisfying the body's energy needs. Some people require modified diets to fulfill special needs: Infants, children, teenagers, and pregnant women require diets that promote growth. People sometimes adjust their eating choices as part of a strategy to gain or lose weight, prevent or control illness, or boost athletic performance.

Elements of a Healthful Diet Your diet supplies CALORIES, or food energy. The number of calories a person needs every day depends on age, size, BODY METABOLISM, and level of physical activity. The average adult man needs about 2,500 calories a day; women generally need fewer. These requirements vary widely, however.

A diet should also supply a full range of NUTRIENTS: proteins, fats, HEALTHY CHOICES carbohydrates, vitamins, minerals, and WATER. A variety of foods—including lean meats, poultry, fish; beans, eggs, and nuts; low-fat dairy products; grain products; and fruits and vegetables—should be consumed to get essential nutrients. Nutritionists advise that in a well-balanced diet, 55 to 60 percent of all calories should come from foods

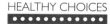

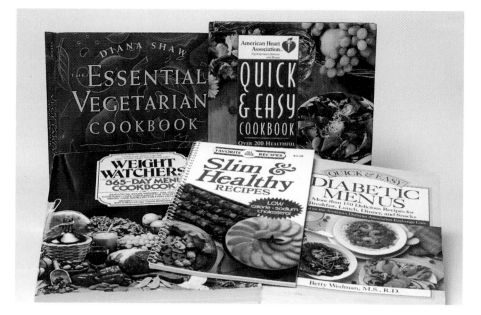

Diets. *Specialized cookbooks can help you enjoy a wide variety of delicious foods, even when you are on a limited diet.*

high in CARBOHYDRATES, no more than 30 percent from FATS, and the remainder from PROTEINS.

Dieting to Lose Weight Losing excess weight (consisting of body fat) may improve physical function and reduce the risk of a variety of diseases. An effective WEIGHT-LOSS STRATEGY reduces the number of calories consumed but retains enough of the nutrients necessary for good health. If you are "dieting" for this purpose, use the FOOD GUIDE PYRAMID as a guide to make sure that daily nutrient recommendations are met and that your FIBER intake is adequate.

Losing weight is easier if your eating plan includes foods you enjoy and satisfies your nutritional needs without causing excessive HUNGER or FATIGUE. Losing weight is also easier and more effective when a lower-calorie diet is combined with regular EXERCISE, or at least moderate physical activity. Regular exercise plus a healthful diet should become habitual in order to keep the weight off. Resist extreme measures to lose weight, and beware of programs that promise quick and easy weight loss. They are often expensive, ineffective, and unhealthful; some are dangerous. Many FAD DIETS cause a loss of muscle tissue. (See also DIET AIDS; DIET FOOD.)

Dieting to Gain Weight If gaining weight is your goal, you will want to gain muscle tissue, not fat. To promote gains in muscle tissue, follow the FOOD GUIDE PYRAMID, but increase the number or size of servings from each food group, eat more frequently, and build muscles with STRENGTH TRAINING. (See also WEIGHT-GAIN STRATEGY.)

Vegetarian Diets A VEGETARIAN DIET excludes all types of meat, poultry, and fish. *Vegans,* or *strict vegetarians,* also exclude eggs and dairy products; they may need DIETARY SUPPLEMENTS to get enough of some of the nutrients found in animal sources. Vegetarians rely on alternative sources for protein, such as beans, nuts, eggs, and cheese. An increasing number of people today are choosing a vegetarian or near-vegetarian diet as a healthful alternative to a traditional meat-centered diet.

HEALTHY CHOICES

RISK FACTORS

HEALTHY CHOICES

Diets for Athletes   An athlete who actively trains and competes may have very high energy needs. Daily calorie requirements for long-distance runners, for example, may be as high as 6,000 calories. Most of this energy—60 to 65 percent—should come from carbohydrates. A high-performance diet of this kind should include lots of *complex carbohydrates* and proteins, and no more than 30 percent of its calories should come from fat. Extra energy expenditure also increases the need for VITAMIN B COMPLEX, which can be provided by eating more vitamin-rich foods. Vitamin B supplements are not needed. Breads and cereals, fruits and vegetables, poultry, fish, and nonfat milk are excellent foods for athletes. Plenty of fluids should also be consumed before, during, and after exercise.

HEALTHY CHOICES
● ● ● ● ● ● ● ● ● ● ● ●

Diets to Treat and Prevent Illness   People who are managing certain health problems or recovering from illness may need special diets. For example, a *bland diet,* one that is especially easy to digest, may be prescribed for someone who has been ill or has a gastrointestinal disorder. A *low-fiber diet* may be recommended for people who have certain digestive disorders. Easily digested foods (such as eggs, milk, cream soups, and cooked vegetables) may be recommended in small amounts at frequent intervals. A *high-fiber diet* may help relieve constipation. It includes plenty of whole-grain breads and cereals as well as raw and stewed fruits and vegetables.

A *low-fat diet* (especially one low in saturated fat) may help lower blood CHOLESTEROL levels in many people, so it is often prescribed for people at risk for atherosclerosis and coronary artery disease. High-fat foods (such as butter, cheese, pastry, nuts, peanut butter, and creamy sauces) are limited, and saturated fat makes up no more than 7 to 10 percent of total calories. A low-fat diet is also advised for patients with gallbladder disease and is believed to reduce the risk of various forms of cancer. A *low-sodium diet,* which restricts salty foods, can help people with kidney or liver disease, high blood pressure, or congestive heart failure.

A *low-purine diet,* consisting of foods low in fat and high in carbohydrates, is advised for people who have gout. Recommended foods include skim milk, fruits, vegetables, and enriched breads and cereals. A *gluten-free diet* helps patients with celiac disease, an inherited disorder in which there is sensitivity to gluten, a protein found in wheat, barley, and rye. Any foods containing these grains must be eliminated from the diet. A *diabetic diet,* important for controlling diabetes mellitus, provides carefully balanced amounts of carbohydrates, protein, and fat. A system of food exchanges supported by the American Diabetes Association makes this diet easier to follow. (See also APPETITE; DIETARY GUIDELINES; EXCHANGE SYSTEM; NUTRITION; PHYTOCHEMICALS; RECOMMENDED DIETARY ALLOWANCES; WEIGHT MANAGEMENT.)

▶ **DIGESTION**

Digestion is the process of breaking down food into simpler substances for use by the body. The end products of digestion are absorbed through the intestinal wall and into the bloodstream and distributed to all the cells of the body for nourishment.

All foods contain NUTRIENTS, which are divided into six types: vitamins, minerals, water, carbohydrates, proteins, and fats. VITAMINS, MINERALS, and WATER are absorbed into the bloodstream without change. Other nutrients in food must be broken down by digestion into simpler elements that the body can use. For example, complex CARBOHYDRATES (starches) are broken down into simple sugars, which the body then uses for energy. PROTEINS are converted to substances that the body uses to repair and replace cells. FATS are changed during digestion to substances that provide energy and store certain vitamins.

How Digestion Works The *digestive system* uses a series of physical and chemical processes. These processes begin in the mouth, where food is ground into smaller pieces and mixed with saliva. Saliva contains a digestive juice that begins to reduce carbohydrates to simple sugars. After the food is swallowed, it moves through the esophagus by means of a series of muscular contractions and enters the stomach. Food is broken into smaller particles by the stomach's churning action. Acids and digestive juices chemically simplify the nutrients. In the small intestine, fluids (bile) produced by the liver and stored in the gallbladder separate fats into smaller particles. Secretions from the pancreas further break down carbohydrates, fats, and proteins. Enzymes produced by the small intestine complete the changes that food undergoes in the digestive system. The products of this process are absorbed through the lining of the small intestine into the bloodstream or lymphatic system. Finally, undigestible matter such as FIBER passes into the large intestine and is expelled as feces.

Digestive Problems Digestion can be disrupted by any problem that affects the breakdown and absorption of nutrients or prevents food from traveling through the digestive system. Examples include congenital abnormalities, infections, vomiting, heartburn, ulcers, inflammatory and autoimmune disorders, tumors, and allergic conditions.

HEALTHY CHOICES
●●●●●●●●●●●●

Maintaining Good Digestion A healthy, well-balanced diet with plenty of fiber helps maintain healthy digestion. Additional LIFESTYLE factors that contribute to good digestion include adequate sleep, regular EXERCISE, drinking enough water, and setting aside a relaxed period for mealtimes. (See also APPETITE; BODY METABOLISM; ENERGY, FOOD; HUNGER; DIGESTIVE SYSTEM, 1.)

▶ **EATING DISORDERS** Eating disorders are health problems characterized by extremely harmful eating patterns. Two common eating disorders are *anorexia* (sometimes called anorexia nervosa) and *bulimia* (also called bulimia nervosa). They are different problems but may arise from the same causes. Sometimes the two conditions are combined, or one may lead to the other.

Both anorexia and bulimia are most common in adolescent girls and young women. Normal changes that occur during adolescence, such as wider hips, cause some girls to become uncomfortable with their bodies and feel that they look too fat. Only a small percentage of people with these disorders are male, although the number is increasing. Both conditions can have damaging effects on the body and may even cause death.

Medical and psychological treatment are usually needed to overcome the abnormal eating patterns typical of these conditions.

Symptoms of Anorexia People with anorexia starve themselves because they have an irrational fear of becoming fat. At the beginning, they may merely go on a weight-loss diet. Soon the idea of losing weight, and the idea of food itself, becomes an obsession. In addition to dieting, people with anorexia may exercise constantly to lose more and more weight. Even when they become extremely thin, they see themselves as fat (see illustration: Distorted Body Image). As a great deal of weight is lost, they feel the physical effects of MALNUTRITION, including FATIGUE. Women with anorexia often stop menstruating and may grow fine body hair called *lanugo*. Self-starvation often leads to heart and kidney disorders. People with anorexia usually also suffer from other psychological problems, including depression. Unless medical help is provided, body weight can drop to a dangerously low level.

Causes and Treatment of Anorexia Anorexia is probably caused by a combination of factors. While the tendency to develop it may be inherited, psychological pressure also seems to bring out the condition. People who have anorexia are often high achievers, typically trying hard to please the people around them. They may also have low self-esteem and an unusually strong fear of growing up.

RISK FACTORS
▶ ▶ ▶ ▶ ▶ ▶

Experts believe that anorexia has a social basis as well. The frequency of the disease has increased greatly in the last 25 to 30 years, an era that has increasingly seen notions of beauty strongly linked with thinness. For example, while the average American woman is 5'4" tall and weighs a healthy 142 pounds, the average fashion model is 5'9" and weighs only 110 pounds. As a result, some people, particularly young women, may become unhappy and feel unattractive when they are not "thin enough."

Treatment of anorexia combines medical care with psychological counseling. Convincing people who have anorexia that they have a problem and are in need of help can be very difficult. Both regaining the lost weight and psychological counseling to break harmful eating patterns are important. Long-term care is usually needed to prevent the problem from returning.

Symptoms of Bulimia Bulimia is a disorder that involves binge eating followed by self-induced vomiting, which can lead to serious physical problems. Like anorexia, bulimia is related to a fear of gaining weight, but the two conditions are different in certain ways. People with bulimia do not necessarily lose as much weight as do those with anorexia. In addition, people with bulimia usually realize that they have a problem that they cannot control.

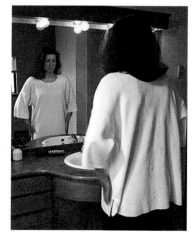

Distorted Body Image. *People with anorexia perceive themselves as "too fat," no matter how thin they really are. They see a distorted image of their bodies and consequently starve themselves to change that image.*

Bulimia often begins with an attempt to diet. When people with bulimia become hungry, they go on an eating binge. They typically consume (usually in secret) large quantities of high-calorie foods in a short time. Then they vomit deliberately, use laxatives, or exercise compulsively in order to "purge" (get rid of) the food and prevent a weight gain. This behavior soon becomes a pattern. Over time, binge eating can cause the stomach to enlarge. Persistent vomiting can cause rashes, swollen ankles and feet, dehydration, rupture of the stomach or esophagus, and tooth damage because of excessive contact with stomach acid.

A related eating disorder is *compulsive overeating,* which involves binging without purging. Compulsive overeating differs from ordinary overeating because compulsive overeaters are not in control of their eating. Unlike most people who overeat, they cannot change their behavior without help. Compulsive overeaters may gain large amounts of weight or may alternate periods of overeating with periods of very strict dieting.

RISK FACTORS
▶ ▶ ▶ ▶ ▶ ▶

Causes and Treatment of Bulimia   Bulimia is often caused by the same factors that lead to anorexia. People with bulimia tend to set very high standards for themselves, but they have low self-esteem. They are troubled by the same social pressures to be thin that cause anorexia, and they have a similar preoccupation with food and eating.

Treatment for bulimia is similar to treatment for anorexia. People with either disorder need a combination of medical care and psychological counseling to break out of the binge eating and vomiting cycle. They often need ongoing support in order to stay well.

CONSULT A
PHYSICIAN

Confronting Eating Disorders   Today there are many sources of help for people with eating disorders. Treatment centers and teams of medical professionals specialize in these conditions. If you think you may have an eating disorder, or if you suspect someone you know of having one, get medical help as early as possible. It may take several attempts to get a person with anorexia to accept help, but it is important to keep trying. Treatment programs can break harmful eating patterns and replace them with healthful eating habits. Counseling can also provide continuing support to prevent the problem from recurring. (See also FASTING; FOOD CRAVING; UNDERWEIGHT; WEIGHT ASSESSMENT; ANOREXIA/BULIMIA, **5.**)

▶ **ENDURANCE**

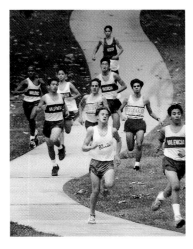

Building Endurance. *Increased cardiovascular endurance is a vital aspect of overall fitness.*

Endurance, or stamina, is the body's ability to perform a prolonged physical activity without tiring. Endurance, STRENGTH, and FLEXIBILITY are the basic elements of physical FITNESS.

Endurance is made up of two components: *cardiovascular endurance* and *muscular endurance.* A strong heart pumps greater amounts of oxygen-rich blood, while strong muscles extract and use oxygen efficiently. The endurance of both the heart and muscles can be increased by regular, prolonged EXERCISE.

Increasing Cardiovascular Endurance   The cardiovascular system—the heart, lungs, and blood vessels—delivers oxygen to all parts of the body, including the muscles. Cardiovascular fitness is increased through regular AEROBIC EXERCISE, such as WALKING, SWIMMING, RUNNING, CYCLING, rowing, sports that require a lot of running, and cross-country skiing. This kind of exercise requires the cardiovascular system to work harder to meet the body's higher oxygen needs. During intense aerobic exercise, the heart rate can rise as much as 400 percent, increasing the amount of blood pumped from 5 quarts (4.7 L) a minute to as many as 20 quarts (19 L) a minute. Regular aerobic exercise builds the heart's endurance by strengthening its walls and enlarging its pumping chamber, increasing the amount of blood pumped with each heartbeat.

Increasing Muscular Endurance   Training increases the number of capillaries in the muscles, so the muscles can receive more blood during exercise. In addition, the activity of certain chemicals called *enzymes* in the muscles increases with exercise and allows muscles to extract and use oxygen more efficiently, also improving muscular endurance.

HEALTHY CHOICES

There are several ways to increase muscular endurance. Regular aerobic exercise (three or four times a week) will help improve endurance for the specific muscles exercised. Running, for example, can greatly improve endurance in the legs but will do little to build endurance in the upper body. Endurance training requires regular workouts that place heavy, repeated demands on muscle groups for progressively longer periods of time. It differs from strength training, which emphasizes the amount of resistance placed against the muscles. Endurance training tends to use less resistance for more repetitions of a given exercise. A recommended training schedule is three times a week, with at least a day of rest between workouts to prevent muscle fatigue, soreness, and injury. (See also STRENGTH TRAINING.)

▶ ENERGY, FOOD

Food energy is the fuel that the human body needs to function. People need energy for every process of living: to breathe, to move, to think, to grow, and to maintain body temperature. They get energy from NUTRIENTS in the food they eat.

How Food Becomes Energy   When you eat food, the CARBOHYDRATES, FATS, and PROTEINS it contains are converted into fuel for your body. GLUCOSE, a type of SUGAR that is the body's primary fuel, is used to produce energy as soon as it enters the bloodstream. *Metabolism* is the process of changing nutrients into energy or into substances that the body can use to build and repair tissues. (See also BODY METABOLISM.)

Food Energy. *Starch is a carbohydrate found in grains and vegetables, and it is the primary energy source in a person's diet.*

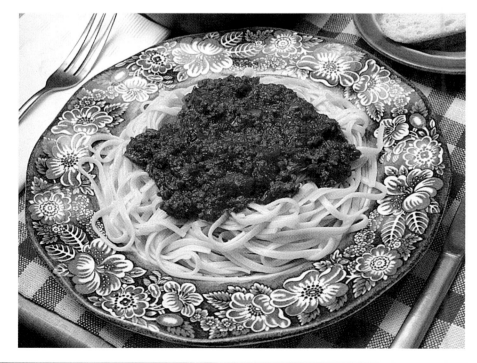

Not all the energy value of food is used immediately. Some is stored for later use. Some glucose is stored in the liver and muscles in the form of *glycogen.* Energy is also stored in the form of fat, some under the skin and some around vital organs. The *fatty acids,* which are combined with glycerol (an oily substance) to form fat, are the body's long-term energy reserve and are available for conversion to energy as needed. (See also LIVER, 1.)

Measuring Food Energy The energy potential of food is measured in units of heat called CALORIES. A food's calorie count is the amount of energy the food provides when metabolized. Proteins and carbohydrates provide 4 calories per gram; a gram of fat provides 9 calories. Therefore, foods that are high in fat tend to contain more calories of food energy than lower-fat foods. On the other hand, WATER and FIBER provide no food energy, so foods containing large amounts of these substances have fewer calories.

When energy, either from body fat or from food, is used by the body, the process is called burning calories. In the long term, a person's weight stability depends on the balance between energy intake (calories consumed) and energy output (calories burned). When intake is greater, weight is gained; when output is greater, weight is lost; and when they are equal, weight is stable. (See also ENERGY, PHYSICAL; WEIGHT MANAGEMENT.)

▶ **ENERGY, PHYSICAL** Physical energy is the body's capacity for doing work. People need physical energy for every action, from running a marathon to keeping their hearts beating. They also need energy to allow their muscles to recover from physical activity.

Energy Used by the Body Physical energy comes from NUTRIENTS in the food we eat and oxygen in the air we breathe. These are converted by the body into the many different chemicals that make up all our cells and body fluids, including the major substances that supply energy: GLUCOSE and BODY FAT. (See also ENERGY, FOOD.)

To generate energy for movement, the body actually relies on instant chemical change within the muscle cells themselves; no substances from outside are needed. After the muscle has contracted and relaxed a few times, however, the chemicals in the cells must be restored to their former state. This is when the energy substances are used, or *burned,* in a relatively slow chemical reaction, during which they are broken down and combined with oxygen. Thus, working muscles need a steady supply not only of oxygen from the blood but also of energy substances from the digestion of food. These substances come chiefly from the CARBOHYDRATES and FATS that we eat, though PROTEINS can also be used as a source of energy. When the body has not digested enough food to produce the needed energy, it uses stored energy in the form of body fat or *glycogen,* a chemical that is formed from GLUCOSE and stored in the liver and muscles.

The energy output of the body is measured in CALORIES, the same units that are used to measure the energy contained in foods. This measurement enables nutritionists to monitor the relationship between diet, exercise, and weight gain or loss.

CALORIES BURNED IN VARIOUS ACTIVITIES			
Activity	Per pound every 10 min.	By a 120-lb person every 10 min.	By a 190-lb person every 10 min.
Bicycling			
Moderate (10 mph)	0.5	60	95
Football (touch)	0.40	48	76
Handball	0.63	76	120
Hiking	0.42	50	80
Judo and karate	0.87	104	165
Running			
10 mph (6 min/mi)	1	120	190
Skiing (snow)			
Downhill	0.59	71	112
Cross-country	0.78	94	148
Soccer	0.63	76	120
Swimming (crawl)			
20 yd/min)	0.32	38	61
Tennis			
Moderate	0.46	55	87
Volleyball	0.36	43	68
Walking			
2 mph	0.22	26	42
Basal metabolism			
Man	0.076	9.1	14
Woman	0.068	8.2	13

Source: Levy, Marvin R., Mark Dignan, and Janet H. Shirreffs. 1992. *Life & health: Targeting wellness.* New York: McGraw-Hill.

Calorie Requirements for Energy   Calorie requirements vary, depending on a person's *basal metabolic rate* and level of physical activity. Basal metabolic rate is the speed at which the body burns calories to handle its basic processes, when it is neither digesting nor involved in exercise. It differs from person to person and is affected by many factors, including weight and BODY COMPOSITION. These factors also affect the number of calories burned in exercise (see chart: Calories Burned in Various Activities). (See also BODY METABOLISM.)

Exercise and basal metabolism affect the number of calories a person needs every day. You do not, however, need highly detailed knowledge of your metabolism to figure out your own energy needs. You can monitor your food intake and body weight during several weeks of typical activity. If your weight remains the same, your energy needs are balanced. (See also EXERCISE; REST; WEIGHT MANAGEMENT.)

▶ **EXCHANGE SYSTEM**   The exchange system is a method of diet planning that groups foods according to the CALORIES and the amounts of NUTRIENTS such as PROTEINS, CARBOHYDRATES, and FATS they contain. Foods within each group can be exchanged for each other. The system is used primarily by people with diabetes, who need to keep track of the calories they consume and the nutrient sources of those calories. However, it can also be useful as a tool to help anyone maintain a balanced diet.

How the System Works   In the exchange system, foods are divided into three main groups, each of which is divided into several smaller groups.

- ▸ The carbohydrate group, which is made up of all foods that are high in carbohydrates, includes the starch, milk, fruit, vegetable, and other carbohydrates groups.
- ▸ The meat and meat substitute group, which consists of foods that are high in protein and low in carbohydrates, is divided into very lean, lean, medium-fat, and high-fat meats and meat substitutes.
- ▸ The fat group, which consists of foods that are high in fats and low in other nutrients, includes saturated, monounsaturated, and polyunsaturated fats.

Each group has a specified serving size called an exchange. For the milk subgroup, for example, an exchange is the equivalent of 1 cup (237 ml) of nonfat milk. Because all foods in the group supply similar amounts of carbohydrates, protein, fat, and calories, one can easily be substituted for another in any meal. For example, one small apple is one fruit exchange. The apple can be exchanged for one large grapefruit half; a whole grapefruit is counted as two fruit exchanges. Foods from one subgroup cannot automatically be substituted for each other, however. For example, although fruits and vegetables are both in the carbohydrate group, they are in different subgroups. Vegetables are lower in carbohydrates than fruits and contain some protein, which fruits do not provide.

There are some differences between the guidelines in the exchange system and those in the FOOD GUIDE PYRAMID. Some of the exchanges are smaller than the servings in the pyramid. A meat exchange, for example, is 1 ounce (28 g). A 3-ounce (85-g) serving of meat would count as three meat exchanges. Also, grouping foods according to their carbohydrate, protein, and fat content brings together foods from different food groups in the pyramid. For example, cheese is in the meat and meat substitutes group in the exchange system because the carbohydrate, protein, and fat content of cheese is similar to that of meat. Bacon and olives are in the fat group because both have very high fat content. These groupings highlight useful nutritional similarities among foods.

Using the System   A diet based on the exchange system would specify the number of exchanges to be chosen daily from each group. For example, a diet of 2,000 calories each day might include 10 starch exchanges, 6 meat exchanges, 4 vegetable exchanges, 5 fruit exchanges, 2 milk exchanges, and 7 fat exchanges. A variety of foods could be selected to meet the exchange totals for the day. The exchange system also includes a list of "free foods" that can be used throughout the day without counting toward the daily number of exchanges. These foods include sugar-free drinks, seasonings, and condiments such as ketchup.

Planning a diet according to the exchange system is a complex process that requires the help of a *dietitian*. The dietitian determines how many calories you should consume daily and how many food exchanges from each group should be consumed in order to obtain those calories. Then, when planning a meal, you must consult lists that show which foods in each group provide the right number of exchanges. Although complicated at first, the exchange system can be useful in regulating diet because it is precise. Most people find that the exchange allowances and groups become familiar when they are used regularly. (See also DIETARY GUIDELINES; DIABETES, 3.)

▷ **EXERCISE**

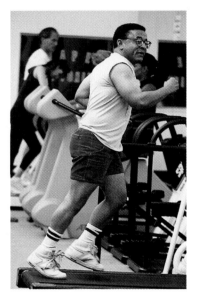

Exercise. *Because many people's daily routines involve little exercise, they need to plan a regular exercise program to stay fit.*

Exercise is physical activity whose purpose is recreation or to promote FITNESS. Although it is often thought of as being separate from the movements and exertions required by work and everyday life, this need not be the case. Making physical activity a regular and enjoyable part of your LIFESTYLE is one of the easiest ways to gain the many benefits of exercise. However, for people whose work and everyday lives tend to be relatively inactive, scheduling regular exercise sessions may be necessary to maintain or improve overall health.

Health and Exercise Adequate levels of activity and movement are necessary to keep the human body fit. Regular exercise is what keeps the body's major components strong and in working order. Exercise also speeds BODY METABOLISM, increasing the rate at which CALORIES are burned.

People who exercise regularly are healthier than those who do not. As a group, they are sick less often and live longer. They experience fewer serious medical conditions and diseases, including heart disease, hypertension, osteoporosis, and even cancer. They have less difficulty managing their weight and therefore avoid the health problems associated with *obesity*.

Exercise has significant psychological benefits as well. It reduces stress and promotes relaxation. People who exercise also tend to have a greater sense of general well-being and higher self-esteem than those who do not.

Any amount of exercise is worthwhile. The Surgeon General's report *Physical Activity and Health,* published in 1996, concluded that 30 minutes of moderate activity each day, such as walking briskly, can provide significant health benefits. This exercise need not be performed all at once: The regular activities of daily living, such as climbing stairs, walking a dog, or bicycling to work can add up to noticeable health gains. However, these modest benefits can be increased with larger amounts of exercise, more varied types of exercise, or more vigorous activities. In general, the greater the amount of exercise, the greater the resulting overall fitness.

Forms of Exercise Any activity that requires a body to move and work can be a form of exercise; the possibilities are endless. One useful way to categorize forms of exercise is by their purpose. Some types of exercise, including many sports, games, and outdoor activities, are intended primarily for recreation. Others, such as riding a stationary bicycle or running on a treadmill, are primarily intended to promote fitness. Still others are lifestyle activities, such as walking or cycling as a mode of transportation. Most forms of exercise, however, serve more than one of these purposes.

Exercise can also be categorized by the demands it places on the heart and lungs and the type of benefits it offers to the body. AEROBIC EXERCISE, such as long-distance running, demands increased supplies of oxygen for extended periods of time. As a result, it increases the HEART RATE and the rate of breathing in order to supply extra oxygen to the body. Aerobic exercises are excellent for improving the health of the cardiovascular system. ANAEROBIC EXERCISE is characterized by short bursts of intensive physical exertion, such as sprinting. These demanding activities require more oxygen than the cardiovascular system can rush to body tissues on a short-term basis and so can be sustained only for a brief time. Anaerobic exercise can be a good way to develop both STRENGTH and muscular ENDURANCE. STRENGTH TRAINING builds stronger muscles, while STRETCHING EXERCISES improve FLEXIBILITY.

Exercise Precautions   Vigorous exercise has its risks, including the possibility of injury. Generally, the more strenuous and demanding the activity, the greater the chances of injury. By taking some basic precautions, however, you can greatly reduce the risks of exercising.

- ▸ Avoid the temptation to do too much too soon. This is especially important if you have not been exercising regularly. For people who are at risk of heart disease, it may be advisable to have a physical examination and a *stress test* before beginning a program of vigorous exercise. (See also STRESS TEST, **3.**)
- ▸ Before performing any demanding exercise, warm up your muscles gradually with a little light exercise; then perform a few stretching exercises to loosen up the joints.
- ▸ When doing strength exercises, do not push your muscles too hard. Increase your *overload,* the maximum effort you demand from your muscles, gradually.
- ▸ Always dress appropriately for the type of exercise you intend to do. Choose exercise clothing that keeps your body at a comfortable temperature. Well-made and well-fitted ATHLETIC FOOTWEAR is especially important for any exercise that puts strain on the feet and knees.
- ▸ Avoid exercising in extremely hot or extremely cold weather.
- ▸ Drink plenty of water before, during, and after exercise sessions to reduce the chances of DEHYDRATION.
- ▸ Pay attention to your body. Stop exercising if you feel breathless, nauseated, or dizzy. If you feel acute pain in your chest or radiating through your shoulder or arm for more than 2 minutes, seek medical attention immediately.
- ▸ Do not eat meals or drink alcohol too soon before an exercise session.

(See also ENERGY, PHYSICAL; EXERCISE AND HEAT INJURY; EXERCISE MACHINES; FITNESS TRAINING; INTERVAL TRAINING; RISK FACTORS; SPORTS AND FITNESS; SPORTS INJURIES; SPORTS NUTRITION; WARM-UP AND COOLDOWN; WEIGHT MANAGEMENT.)

▶ EXERCISE AND HEAT INJURY

A variety of health problems can result from EXERCISE in hot or humid weather. When air temperature approaches body temperature, or when high humidity saturates the air with water, the body is less able to cool itself adequately. Direct sunlight on the skin may also raise body heat. An overheated body is vulnerable to several heat-related medical problems, including dehydration, heat cramps, heat exhaustion, and heatstroke.

Exercise and Body Temperature   During exercise, the body's heat production increases to as much as 20 times the normal rate. The body gets rid of this excess heat through *perspiration,* or by sweating. Sweat consists of WATER, SALTS, and other substances that are excreted through glands in the skin. As sweat evaporates from the skin, it takes heat away from the body. Perspiration normally results in a loss of between 12 and 24 ounces (about 350 to 700 ml) of water each day. During hot weather and vigorous exercise, however, this amount can increase to 1 quart (about 1 L) or more per hour. Even during cold weather, strenuous exercise can cause heavy perspiration.

RISK FACTORS
▶ ▶ ▶ ▶ ▶ ▶

Problems Caused by Heat   The body's cooling system is most efficient when the air is dry; humidity makes evaporation more difficult. Exercising in hot or humid weather may bring on *heat cramps,* painful muscle spasms that are caused by an imbalance of fluids and salts in the body. Heat cramps may occur during or after a workout.

Heat exhaustion is a more serious problem that results from a heavy loss of fluids and salts due to profuse sweating. This severe form of DEHYDRATION can cause cold, pale, clammy skin; FATIGUE; rapid heartbeat; weakness; and dizziness. To relieve these symptoms, stop exercising; rest in a cool, dry place; and drink large amounts of cool liquids to bring your temperature down. A cool bath or shower may also be helpful.

Untreated heat exhaustion may progress to *heatstroke,* an acute medical emergency that occurs when the body's cooling mechanisms break down completely so that body temperature rises rapidly. Heatstroke may

Working Out in the Heat.
Coaches of organized sports have to monitor weather conditions during summer workouts and be attentive to signs of heat-related problems in their athletes.

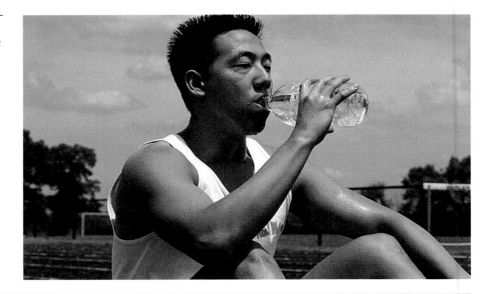

be caused by strenuous exercise in hot or humid weather. One of the first symptoms of heatstroke is that sweating stops and the skin becomes dry and very hot. Lacking the cooling effect of perspiration, body temperature can rise quickly to 106°F (41.1°C) or more. This excessive body temperature can harm the brain, heart, and other organs. Other symptoms of heatstroke include grogginess, confusion, collapse, and—eventually—coma. Low levels of body fluids may upset blood chemistry, leading to kidney failure, liver damage, and blood clotting abnormalities.

CONSULT A
PHYSICIAN

Heatstroke requires immediate medical treatment. Until assistance arrives, a person suspected of having heatstroke should be moved out of the sun into a cool place and have cold compresses or ice packs applied to the body. (See also HEATSTROKE, **8.**)

Preventing Heat-Related Problems   The key to preventing heat-related sports problems is to use common sense when exercising in weather that is significantly hotter or more humid than you are used to. First, it is essential to drink liquids before, during, and after any hot-weather workout to replace the fluid you expect to lose in sweating. Normally, your sense of *thirst* prompts the replacement of lost fluids, but during hot weather or intense exercise, your body's response may lag far behind its actual need for water. Therefore, you must make a conscious effort to drink plenty of fluids. Water is sufficient, although some people prefer specially prepared sports drinks, which replace other substances lost through sweating. (See also BEVERAGES; SPORTS NUTRITION.) As a general rule, drink at least 2 cups (about 0.5 L) of water, juice, milk, or a sports drink a couple of hours before a sports activity. Just before participating, drink 2 more cups (about 0.5 L) of water or a sports drink. During and after the activity, try to drink $\frac{1}{2}$ cup (about 118 ml) of water or a sports drink every 15 minutes. Increase these amounts in very hot weather.

HEALTHY CHOICES
●●●●●●●●●●●●

Second, stay alert to the early symptoms of heat-related problems. A serious medical condition can develop quickly. In hot weather, an exercise such as SWIMMING that is unlikely to produce overheating may be preferred. However, if you choose to run or play tennis when it is hot, it may be wise to shorten your workout or to exercise during the cooler early morning or evening hours.

▶ EXERCISE MACHINES

Exercise machines can be used in a variety of ways to enhance fitness, whether at a gym or at home. Each type of machine has its own particular advantages. Some, such as stationary bicycles and treadmills, provide an excellent way to get AEROBIC EXERCISE. Others, such as weight machines, are used primarily to build muscle STRENGTH. Used in combination, or properly coordinated with other forms of regular EXERCISE, these machines can be a valuable part of an overall FITNESS program. All of them offer the advantage of indoor use regardless of outside weather.

Stationary Bicycles   The most popular home exercise machine is the stationary bike. Bicycling in place on such a machine makes an excellent

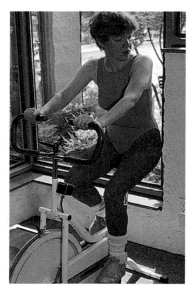

Stationary Bike. *A stationary bike is a relatively affordable machine that can be used at home. It offers a variety of workout benefits, such as increased muscular endurance, strength, and cardiovascular conditioning.*

Exercise Equipment. *A fitness center or gym has a wide range of machines that make it possible to plan an exercise program that best suits individual needs.*

aerobic workout; the machine also builds leg strength and endurance by providing *resistance* as you pedal. Machines that allow for arm movement while pedaling help build upper-body strength as well. A good stationary bike has a sturdy frame, a comfortable seat, smooth pedaling action, and simple controls for adjusting the level of resistance. Some models include ergometers, devices that measure the amount of work done, sometimes in terms of calories burned. These are not necessary, however, because you can use your HEART RATE and a clock to measure the effectiveness of your workout and your progress from session to session.

Rowing Machines   By duplicating the action of rowing a boat, a rowing machine combines an aerobic workout with strength and endurance training for the major muscles of the back, arms, shoulders, and legs. Most rowing machines use adjustable hydraulic pistons to produce resistance. Look for a sturdy model that has a sliding seat, smooth action, and convenient, adjustable controls.

Cross-Country Ski Machines   Another popular type of exercise machine simulates cross-country skiing. A ski machine develops aerobic conditioning, endurance in arm and leg muscles, coordination, and FLEXIBILITY. This device has short skis on rollers, with cables or poles for the arms. Many models have adjustable resistance for both arms and legs. As with other exercise machines, sturdiness, smooth action, and easy-to-use controls are key features.

Treadmills and Stair-Climbers   Treadmills are machines that allow you to walk or run in place. Although the best kind of treadmill is motorized to move the tread at varying speeds, it has the disadvantage of being expensive and bulky. Treadmills offer a cardiovascular workout and

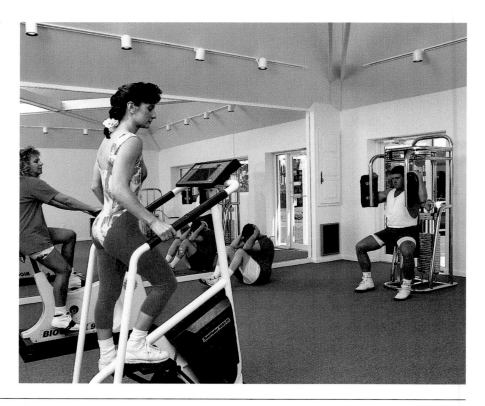

endurance training for leg muscles. These benefits, however, can be duplicated by jogging in place. Stair-climbing machines are a variation of the treadmill that simulates climbing steps, but again, the benefit can also be achieved by climbing actual flights of stairs.

Weight Machines Weight machines such as Nautilus, Cybex, and Universal, also called *resistance equipment,* can be used to exercise all the major muscle groups in the body to increase strength and flexibility. These types of machines are found in most fitness centers. Have an instructor help you when you use weight machines for the first time.

Many of the benefits of weight machines are similar to those of free weights. Free weights, however, have the added advantage of improving coordination and balance as you lift and hold the weights overhead. (See also CROSS TRAINING; ENDURANCE; FITNESS TRAINING; WEIGHT TRAINING.)

▶ FAD DIETS

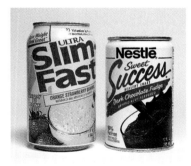

Fad Diets. *Most fad diets are likely to result in weight rebound because they do nothing to improve the eating habits and sedentary lifestyles that led to the excessive weight in the first place.*

A fad diet is any weight-loss diet that is nutritionally unsound. Most fad diets promise quick results. Although they often produce considerable weight loss at the outset, much of that weight is water. These diets are generally ineffective in the long term because any weight that is lost is usually gained back again. Some fad diets are dangerous and have caused serious illnesses and even death.

One type of fad diet is a *liquid diet,* which replaces all or most food with a specially formulated beverage. In the 1970s, a high-protein liquid diet apparently caused 58 people to die suddenly from heart rhythm problems. Although the formulas of liquid diets have been improved, most are intended only for consumption by the very obese: people who are at least 30 percent OVERWEIGHT. These diets are to be followed under the strict supervision of a doctor. Although the widely available diet powders used at home are safe if the person consumes at least one well-balanced meal a day along with plenty of water, these diets are largely ineffective. Most people gain the weight back.

Another example of a fad diet is any diet that severely restricts or eliminates a food group or major nutrient. One such diet is a high-protein, low-carbohydrate diet that was popular for several years. This type of diet is not healthy; it tends to be high in fat and can result in high levels of blood CHOLESTEROL, abnormal heart rhythms, and excessive strain on the kidneys. Other fad diets are restricted to only one or two foods, such as a grapefruit diet or a yogurt diet. *Crash diets,* which provide very few calories, are a particularly dangerous type of fad diet. Followed for too long, they can cause MALNUTRITION or DEHYDRATION.

Losing and gaining weight in cycles, the so-called *yo-yo syndrome,* is a problem for many people. In the yo-yo syndrome, weight loss is often rapid at first. Later, however, the reduced caloric intake causes the *metabolic rate* to slow down so that food energy is conserved by the body. Because the body is using food at a slower rate, weight loss through dieting becomes increasingly difficult. When the fad diet is abandoned, the slower metabolic rate results in a rapid weight gain. Often, the person ends up weighing more than he or she weighed before the diet.

As an effective WEIGHT-LOSS STRATEGY, nutritionists and physicians recommend a well-balanced diet that produces a slow and steady weight loss of 1 to 2 pounds per week. Calories should not be cut to less than 1,600 each day except under a doctor's supervision. A regular EXERCISE program will also help burn fat and increase the metabolic rate. A lifelong change in habits is necessary to eliminate the unhealthy eating practices that lead to excessive weight gain. (See also DIET AIDS; DIETS; FASTING; WEIGHT MANAGEMENT.)

► FAST FOOD

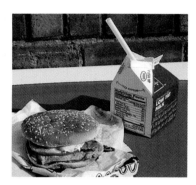

Fast Food. *When eating fast food, choose one of the lower-fat menu items now available at many major fast-food restaurants.*

Fast food is mass-produced food that is served ready to eat at restaurants and food stands. Fast-food restaurants are popular because they provide food quickly and conveniently, often for less money than in traditional restaurants. Typical fast food includes hamburgers, french fries, pizza, fried chicken, hot dogs, and tacos. Many fast foods are high in CALORIES as well as FATS, SALT, and SUGAR, but most are low in other NUTRIENTS. However, fast-food restaurants have made an effort in recent years to offer more nutritious food selections.

A survey by the Food Marketing Institute found that when buying takeout food, nearly half of Americans (48 percent) choose fast-food restaurants over other restaurants or supermarkets. Although fast foods typically supply ample amounts of CARBOHYDRATES and PROTEINS, many are low in vitamins and minerals and extremely high in fats. For example, fat can make up nearly 50 percent of the calories in fried chicken or fish because of cooking oils trapped in the breading. Hamburgers, cheeseburgers, and french fries are also very high in fat; in addition, many fast-food "shakes" are made with vegetable oils instead of milk, adding even more fat. Even green salads and coleslaw can be high in fat because of the mayonnaise or heavy, oily dressings used on them. As a result, some fast foods are so high in calories that they provide for as much as half of an average person's daily calorie needs.

It is possible, however, to make healthy choices when you eat at a fast-food restaurant. Look for foods that are nutritious and low in calories, such as a plain salad, grilled chicken, a plain baked potato, a slice of cheese pizza, a roast beef sandwich, or a bean burrito. Some fast-food restaurants have added salad and pasta bars that allow you to create your own nutritious meal. Most fast-food chains now provide printed nutrition information about their menu items to help you make informed choices. (See also FATS, OILS, AND SWEETS.)

► FASTING

Fasting is deliberately abstaining from food for a period of time. It is required before some medical tests and procedures, and it is part of some religious observances. It is not recommended as a way of losing weight, and it can be dangerous.

The effect of prolonged fasting on the body is the same as starvation. When there is no energy available from food, the body turns to its own tissues for fuel. Reserves of carbohydrates are used first; then fat and muscle tissue is broken down. The rate of BODY METABOLISM slows to conserve energy. The body's resistance to infection is lowered, and the heart may be damaged. The digestive process may slow or stop entirely, and the production of sex hormones shuts down.

As fasting continues, weight loss slows because of the decreased metabolic rate and because the body begins to conserve salt, causing water to be retained in the tissues. Prolonged fasting has health hazards that disqualify it as a weight-control method. In general, a person should not fast for more than a day without medical supervision. (See also FAD DIETS; WEIGHT-LOSS STRATEGY.)

▶ FAT

see BODY FAT; FATS

▶ FATIGUE

Fatigue is a feeling of weariness or tiredness. Fatigue can be caused by lack of sleep, inadequate diet, physical or mental exertion, or psychological factors. Fatigue can also be a symptom of many kinds of illnesses.

Types of Fatigue   Many types of fatigue originate in physical aspects of your LIFESTYLE. Your sleep habits, diet, work or study habits, and physical activities can contribute to fatigue. Most fatigue that has a basis in your lifestyle is normal and healthy; it is usually merely a signal that you need REST.

Fatigue may also have a psychological basis. Conflicts, stress, or boredom can lead to weariness. Physical or mental illness may cause

Fatigue. *A fit person will recover quickly from the fatigue caused by a vigorous workout.*

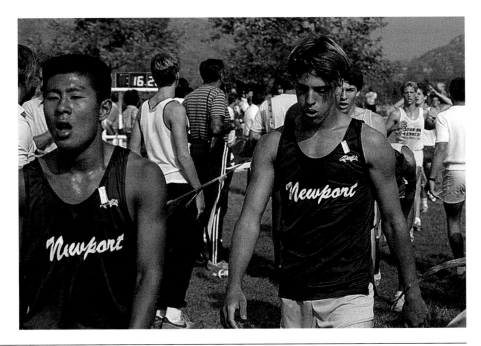

fatigue as well. Physical sicknesses ranging from flu to serious diseases such as anemia or diabetes can all make people feel very tired. Likewise, mental illness such as severe depression or anxiety can cause fatigue.

Symptoms of Fatigue   Physical symptoms of fatigue include body weariness, aching muscles, a loss of coordination, and difficulty in performing physical tasks. Fatigue can also affect mental function, making it difficult to concentrate or make decisions. Fatigue should not be chronic. If it persists, a physician or psychiatrist should be consulted.

CONSULT A
PHYSICIAN

HEALTHY CHOICES
••••••••••

How to Overcome Fatigue   Ordinarily, fatigue can be simply overcome by getting rest or sleep. It may help to change your diet if you are not receiving sufficient food energy. Fatigue that has a psychological basis is more difficult to overcome. People who are fatigued need to try to determine its cause so that they may take appropriate steps to resolve it; doing so often requires psychological counseling. If a person cannot pinpoint the cause of fatigue, implementing a new routine or changing lifestyle habits can help. (See also DEHYDRATION; ENERGY, PHYSICAL; MALNUTRITION; SLEEP, 1; ANEMIA, 3; CHRONIC FATIGUE SYNDROME, 3.)

► FATS

Fats are one of the three *macronutrients,* classes of nutrients that the body needs in large amounts. Fats serve many functions: They provide the body with its most concentrated form of energy; they are an important part of cell membranes; and as BODY FAT, they cushion kidneys and other internal

FAT CONTENT OF FOODS			
Food	**Saturated fat (g)**	**Monounsaturated fat (g)**	**Polyunsaturated fat (g)**
Cheddar cheese (1 oz)	6.0	2.7	0.3
Mozzarella, part skim (1 oz)	3.1	1.4	0.1
Whole milk (1 cup)	5.1	2.4	0.3
Skim milk (1 cup)	0.3	0.1	—
Butter (1 tbsp)	7.1	3.3	0.4
Mayonnaise (1 tbsp)	1.7	3.2	5.8
Tuna in oil (3 oz)	1.4	1.9	3.1
Tuna in water (3 oz)	0.3	0.2	0.3
Lean ground beef, broiled (3 oz)	6.2	6.9	0.6
Leg of lamb, roasted (3 oz)	5.6	4.9	0.8
Bacon (3 slices)	3.3	4.5	1.1
Chicken breast, roasted (3 oz)	0.9	1.1	0.7

Source: U.S. Department of Agriculture.

organs against sudden shock and insulate the body against loss of body heat. Fats also transport vitamins A, D, E, and K throughout the body.

Fats are found in varying concentrations in a wide range of foods (see chart: Fat Content of Foods). Measured in CALORIES, fats generate an average of 9 calories per gram as compared with the 4 calories per gram found in carbohydrates and proteins. This is what makes fats the most "fattening" foods to eat.

Although fats can create problems nutritionally, they are just as essential in the right amounts as PROTEINS and CARBOHYDRATES, the other macronutrients. Fats provide the body with a large, long-term energy reserve, whereas reserves of carbohydrate energy are limited and can soon be exhausted.

Saturated Fats The structure of dietary fats is determined by the number of hydrogen atoms that are attached to the carbon atoms of the fat molecule. Differing types of fats have different effects on health. Saturated fats have the maximum number of hydrogen atoms attached to each molecule. Generally, saturated fats are solid at room temperature. The amount of saturated fat in the diet should be limited because this type of fat contributes to high blood cholesterol levels. A high level of CHOLESTEROL in the blood increases the risk of blocked arteries and atherosclerosis, coronary artery disease, and stroke. Most saturated fats come from animal sources; these include butter, milk fat, and the fat found in meats. Among vegetable fats, coconut and palm oils are also highly saturated. (See also ATHEROSCLEROSIS, **3**; HEART DISEASE, **3**.)

RISK FACTORS
▶ ▶ ▶ ▶ ▶ ▶

Unsaturated Fats Unsaturated fats are not linked up with all the hydrogen atoms they can carry. Depending on how many slots for hydrogen atoms remain open, they are either monounsaturated (with one hydrogen atom missing) or polyunsaturated (with several missing). Unsaturated fats are usually liquid at room temperature. Monounsaturated fats can help lower blood cholesterol levels, perhaps by helping the body to excrete cholesterol. Some of the largely monounsaturated fats are peanut, avocado, and olive oils. Examples of mainly polyunsaturated fats are corn, sesame, and safflower oils. In order to make the unsaturated fats in margarines and shortenings harder and more stable, manufacturers add hydrogen atoms by a process called *hydrogenation*. Unsaturated fats that are hydrogenated, however, pose the same nutritional problems as saturated fats.

Dietary Guidelines Most Americans consume too much fat. On average, about 34 percent of their daily calories come from fats. According to most nutrition experts, people should consume no more than 30 percent of their total calories in the form of dietary fats. Of this 30 percent, it is recommended that no more than 10 percent of total calories come from saturated fats. You can control your fat intake by cutting down on red meat, switching to low-fat dairy products, and avoiding fried foods. Saturated fat consumption can be reduced by using margarine made from corn, safflower, or sunflower oil instead of butter. A rule of thumb used to evaluate saturated fat content is: If it flies, swims, or grows in the ground, it is lower in saturated fat. (See also ENERGY, FOOD; FAST FOOD; FATS, OILS, AND SWEETS; NUTRIENTS; OVERWEIGHT.)

HEALTHY CHOICES
• • • • • • • • • • • •

▶ FATS, OILS, AND SWEETS

Fats, oils, and sweets are a class of foods that are filling and often high in CALORIES but low in valuable NUTRIENTS. Foods in this group include butter, margarine, cooking oil, mayonnaise, sugar, jam, candy, and soft drinks. These foods are high in FATS, SUGAR, or both.

Everyone needs some fats in his or her diet. Fats help keep the skin and hair healthy, transport certain VITAMINS through the body, and produce energy. The relatively small amounts of fat you need, however, are easily obtained from other, more nutritious foods, especially from the MILK, YOGURT, AND CHEESE GROUP and the MEAT, POULTRY, FISH, DRY BEANS, EGGS, AND NUTS GROUP. Many foods classed as fats, oils, and sweets are high in saturated fats and CHOLESTEROL. *Saturated fats* are found mostly in foods that come from animals, and cholesterol is found only in animal products. High levels of saturated fats and cholesterol in the diet increase a person's risk of heart disease and atherosclerosis. Some studies have found links between diets high in fat and the incidence of certain kinds of cancer, especially breast cancer and colorectal cancer. In addition, because fats, oils, and sweets are so high in calories, they often produce an undesired weight gain that leads to *obesity* and the health problems related to it.

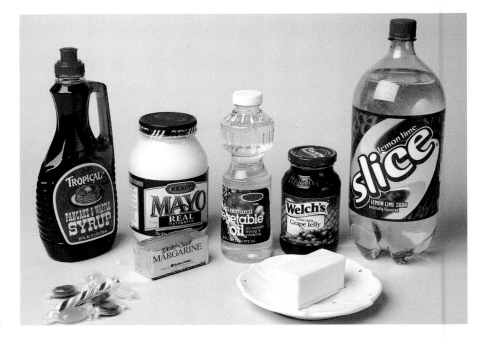

Fats, Oils, and Sweets. *Eat only small amounts of these foods, and never substitute them for more nutritious foods.*

HEALTHY CHOICES

Fats, oils, and sweets are found at the tip of the FOOD GUIDE PYRAMID. Foods in this category should be consumed sparingly. To make fats, oils, and sweets part of a healthy diet, use small amounts to enhance the flavor of the foods you eat from the other food groups. For example, add a pat of butter to broccoli (from the VEGETABLE GROUP), a teaspoon of jam to toast (from the BREAD, CEREAL, RICE, AND PASTA GROUP), or some powdered sugar to fruit salad (from the FRUIT GROUP). There is no need to eliminate fats, oils, and sweets from your diet as long as you enjoy them in moderation and avoid substituting them for foods that are more nutritious. (See also DIETARY GUIDELINES; EXCHANGE SYSTEM; ATHEROSCLEROSIS, **3**; BREAST CANCER, **3**; COLORECTAL CANCER, **3**; HEART DISEASE, **3**.)

▶ FIBER

Fiber, or roughage, is the undigestible part of foods of plant origin. Fiber is a complex CARBOHYDRATE, but unlike other carbohydrates, it is not a NUTRIENT because it does not produce energy for the body. It is an important dietary component, however, because it aids DIGESTION. Foods high in fiber include whole grains, apples, beans, peas, corn, potatoes, and broccoli. Meat and dairy products do not contain fiber.

Types of Fiber   There are two kinds of fiber: soluble and insoluble. *Soluble fiber* dissolves in water. Oat bran and the gummy fibers found in fruits (such as pectin, gums, and mucilages) are soluble. *Insoluble fibers* (cellulose, hemicellulose, and lignin) make up the cell walls of plants. Most foods that contain fiber include both types.

FIBER CONTENT OF SELECTED FOODS	
Food	**Dietary fiber (g)**
Bagel (1 medium)	1
Whole-wheat bread (1 slice)	2
Apple, with skin (1 medium)	3
Pear, with skin (1 medium)	4
Broccoli, cooked (½ cup)	2
Carrot, raw (1 medium)	2
Kidney beans, cooked (½ cup)	3
Popcorn, air-popped (1 cup)	1

Function and Value of Fiber   As fiber passes through the large intestine, it absorbs large amounts of water and binds with digestive waste products. This process creates large, soft stools that move through the digestive tract faster and are easier to eliminate. Some research has associated a high-fiber diet with a lower risk of developing colon cancer, diabetes, and some disorders of the colon such as diverticulitis, constipation, and hemorrhoids. A diet high in fiber can also help people lose weight by filling the stomach without adding CALORIES. Not only does fiber itself contain no calories, but most high-fiber foods are low in calories and FATS. They also tend to be high in VITAMINS and MINERALS.

HEALTHY CHOICES
●●●●●●●●●●●●

Insoluble fiber is more beneficial to the health of the lower digestive tract than soluble fiber. Soluble fiber, however, may help prevent heart disease by lowering the amount of CHOLESTEROL in the bloodstream. Some studies have also found that soluble fiber may help regulate blood sugar levels by slowing the digestion of carbohydrates.

Although nutritionists recommend that people eat 20 to 35 grams of fiber a day, the average American's diet includes only 11 grams of fiber. You can increase fiber intake by eating a high-fiber bran cereal for breakfast and by consuming a variety of fruits and vegetables during the course of the day. Whole-grain breads in place of white bread, as well as nuts and

HEALTHY CHOICES
●●●●●●●●●●●●

seeds such as sunflower seeds, will also add fiber to your diet (see chart: Fiber Content of Selected Foods). (See also DIETARY GUIDELINES.)

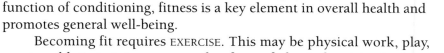

▶ FITNESS

HEALTHY CHOICES
●●●●●●●●●●●●

Fitness is the body's ability to meet the varied physical demands of life. A function of conditioning, fitness is a key element in overall health and promotes general well-being.

Becoming fit requires EXERCISE. This may be physical work, play, sports, athletic training, or any other form of physical activity. In the past, when work was more often physical, the daily LIFESTYLES of most people typically required much more activity than is usual now, assuring a higher level of fitness. In the United States today, fitness levels have consequently declined, creating a serious health problem.

Eating a good diet and getting the right kind and amount of exercise are essential to becoming fit. For those who eat too much or get too little exercise, a commitment to fitness requires significant lifestyle changes.

Fitness can be broken down in several ways. One useful way to think of fitness is to view it as having three primary components: strength, endurance, and flexibility. An additional aspect of fitness is body composition, the proportion of fat to lean tissue in the body.

Strength   STRENGTH most commonly refers to *muscle strength*. It is the amount of force that muscles can exert when they contract. Muscle strength is necessary for all movement, which is created by the contraction of specific muscle groups. Strong muscles allow the body to move more efficiently and do more work. They also help support and protect many of the systems of the body, such as the joints and internal organs. Muscle strength can be improved with STRENGTH TRAINING, which builds muscles by systematically requiring them to do greater amounts of work.

A strong heart is also necessary for fitness. A heart that is strong beats more vigorously and can pump more blood, an essential part of cardiovascular health. *Bone strength* is also important. Although more difficult to measure than muscle strength, bone strength is primarily determined by the density of bone mass. This can be improved with weight-bearing exercises, such as RUNNING.

Endurance   ENDURANCE is the body's ability to sustain an activity or continue to perform work. *Muscular endurance* and *cardiovascular endurance* are the main components. Both are improved through regular AEROBIC EXERCISE, which requires the skeletal muscles, heart, vascular system, and lungs to work hard for prolonged periods. They respond to such exercise by becoming stronger and working hard for progressively greater lengths of time.

Flexibility   The body's ability to move through a full *range of motion*, called FLEXIBILITY, is also an essential component of fitness. Anyone who has experienced stiff, tight muscles or a severe sprain knows how a restricted range of motion limits activity. Flexibility allows muscles and joints to move to their maximum extent, easing all movement and

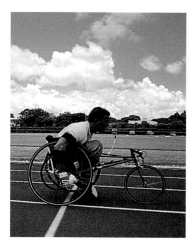

Fitness and Aerobic Exercise.
People of differing abilities can all improve their total fitness through regular exercise.

reducing the risk of injury. Flexibility is improved through STRETCHING EXERCISES that keep muscles supple and loose.

Body Composition Another aspect of fitness is BODY COMPOSITION, the ratio of fat to bone and muscle in the body. A fit person has the appropriate amount of body fat required to maintain good health. People whose body weight has higher percentages of fat should start a FITNESS TRAINING program, whether they are OVERWEIGHT or not.

In general, any exercise that increases strength and endurance is likely to improve body composition by adding muscle mass and increasing energy expenditures. Burning more CALORIES than are consumed requires the body to convert its surplus fat in order to produce the additional energy it requires. (See also SPORTS AND FITNESS; WEIGHT ASSESSMENT.)

▶ FITNESS CENTER

A fitness center is a facility equipped to provide opportunities for EXERCISE and FITNESS TRAINING. Fitness centers vary widely in size, equipment, and staffing. The term may refer to a large area within a building or to a spacious, all-inclusive health club complex.

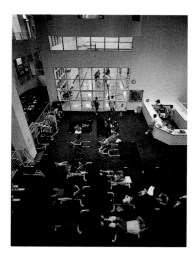

Fitness Center. *For some people, membership in a fitness center provides the motivation to exercise regularly.*

Equipment and Facilities Fitness centers generally offer a variety of EXERCISE MACHINES and other equipment, ranging from treadmills and stair-climbers to weight machines and free weights. In addition, large fitness centers may include such facilities as a swimming pool, a sauna, tennis and racquetball courts, and even a restaurant. A fitness center may also have a library of books and videotapes dealing with health and fitness. Besides instructors, the staff of a fitness center may include PERSONAL TRAINERS, nutritionists, and massage therapists.

Benefits and Drawbacks A large fitness center gives its members an opportunity to take part in various exercise activities and training programs. Members may use many different EXERCISE MACHINES that would be costly to buy. They also have the benefit of staff supervision and instruction. In addition, fitness centers offer their members companionship while they are exercising.

Fitness centers can, however, be expensive to join. As many as half of the people who do join such facilities lose interest within a few months. Fitness centers also vary considerably in quality. Anyone who is thinking of joining a center should find out whether its staff members are certified by the American College of Sports Medicine, the Aerobics and Fitness Association of America, or a similar organization. (See also NUTRITIONIST, **9.**)

▶ FITNESS TRAINING

Fitness training is physical EXERCISE intended to improve a person's overall level of FITNESS. Its goal is to enhance each of the elements of fitness: STRENGTH, ENDURANCE, FLEXIBILITY, and BODY COMPOSITION. Fitness training offers many benefits to your health. Fit people generally feel better, get fewer illnesses and diseases, and live longer. They also gain

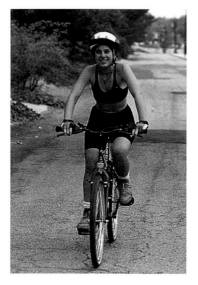

Fitness Training. *To become fit, you must exercise frequently, with enough intensity, and for a sufficient length of time.*

HEALTHY CHOICES
● ● ● ● ● ● ● ● ● ● ● ●

an improved appearance and self-image, extra energy and strength, and reduced fatigue and tension.

Planning a Fitness Program   The particular nature of a fitness program depends on a person's level of fitness and individual goals. In general, however, fitness training involves three major classes of exercise. AEROBIC EXERCISE, such as RUNNING or AEROBIC DANCE, builds endurance by raising the HEART RATE for extended periods of time. It is of special benefit to the cardiovascular system. It can also increase muscle strength and, by burning calories rapidly, improve body composition.

STRENGTH TRAINING, such as weight lifting or working on EXERCISE MACHINES, is primarily intended to build *muscle strength*. Some types of strength training also strengthen bones, improve endurance, and, by adding muscle mass, enhance body composition. STRETCHING EXERCISE is primarily intended to enhance flexibility by expanding the *range of motion* of joints and muscles. It also helps prevent injury, soreness, and stiffness when performed as part of an exercise session.

A good all-around fitness training program for most people combines 3 to 5 sessions of aerobic exercise plus stretching with 2 to 3 sessions of strength training each week. Aerobic workouts and strength workouts can be on the same day or on different days. However, at least 1 day a week should be set aside for REST to allow the body to recover from the demands of exercise.

Achieving Fitness   Improving fitness takes time. When you begin a training program, you may feel some soreness and FATIGUE at first. To minimize these problems, increase the demands you make on your body gradually. *Overload* is defined as the amount you push your body beyond its normal limits. You should increase your overload by no more than 10 percent each week. This change can come from an increase in the frequency, intensity, or duration of your workouts. If you continue to experience symptoms of strain, however, do not increase your overload at all until they subside.

Most people begin feeling more fit in about 6 weeks; they find that they can exercise harder, longer, and more easily than at the start. After 2 to 3 months of regular training, many reach a plateau and will have to work harder to improve aerobic capacity and strength. Keep in mind that if you stop fitness training, fitness gains will be lost in about the same time it took to achieve them. (See also CROSS TRAINING; ENERGY, PHYSICAL; SPORTS AND FITNESS.)

► **FLEXIBILITY**

Flexibility is the ability of joints to move through a full range of motion. Flexibility, STRENGTH, and muscular and cardiovascular ENDURANCE are the basic elements of physical FITNESS. Flexibility is increased when muscles and other connective tissues that support the joints are developed and lengthened with STRETCHING EXERCISES, performed regularly. The elasticity of the connective tissue at each joint also determines flexibility.

The maximum range of motion of body joints varies according to the type of joint. The knee, for example, has a more limited range of

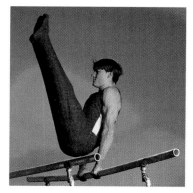

Flexibility. *Gymnasts have a high degree of flexibility.*

motion than the shoulder. However, the flexibility of all joints and muscles can be improved through regular EXERCISE.

Importance of Flexibility Improved flexibility protects against muscle pulls and tears. It also helps in the performance of everyday activities, contributing to better posture, more graceful movement, and fewer aches and pains in joints and muscles. Lower-back pain, for example, can often be reduced by exercises that increase the flexibility of thigh and lower-back muscles while strengthening the abdominal muscles.

Building Flexibility Stretching exercises are the main method of improving flexibility. When beginning a stretching program, exercise muscles slowly and steadily. Maintain a regular routine that progresses gradually. Do not stretch muscles to the point of feeling pain. (See also FITNESS TRAINING; SPORTS INJURIES; STRENGTH TRAINING.)

▶ FOOD ADDITIVES

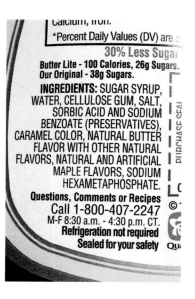

Food Additives. *Food additives are present in many packaged foods, and serve many purposes, including preservation, flavoring, and coloring.*

Food additives are chemical substances added to foods for a variety of purposes. These purposes include preserving food so that it will keep its attractive appearance and freshness longer, boosting nutritional value, improving taste and texture, and adding desired color. In the United States, the Food and Drug Administration (FDA) regulates the use of food additives and has approved about 2,800 different natural and synthetic materials that are used in food preparation.

Preservatives Some preservatives are chemicals called *antimicrobials* that resist the growth of harmful organisms; others are chemicals called *antioxidants* that slow down changes in food color and flavor caused by exposure to air. The most familiar and widely used antimicrobials are SALT and SUGAR. Salt is used to preserve meat and fish, and sugar is used in jam and jelly. Other antimicrobials are calcium propionate, used to keep bread and other baked goods fresh; potassium sorbate and sorbic acid, which are added to processed cheeses, syrups, and margarine; and sodium nitrite, which is used to protect hot dogs and other cured meats from dangerous bacteria, including the organism that causes *botulism*. Common antioxidants are *vitamin C* (ascorbic acid), added to fruit products and acidic foods; BHT, used in products such as cereals and salad dressings; and *vitamin E*, used in vegetable oils.

Nutrition Boosters NUTRIENTS are added to some foods to improve their nutritional value. *Enriched* foods are foods that have lost certain nutrients during processing (for example, white flour) and then had those nutrients added back in. *Fortified* foods, by contrast, have had nutrients added to them that were not present originally. Salt is often fortified with iodide, dairy products with vitamins A and D, orange juice with calcium, and grain products with the B vitamin folic acid.

Flavoring Agents Flavoring agents are used in foods to enhance or change flavor. ARTIFICIAL SWEETENERS such as aspartame are used to sweeten many DIET FOODS. *Monosodium glutamate* (MSG), although it has no taste of its own, is used to enhance the flavor of foods.

Emulsifiers Emulsifiers are used to improve the consistencies of foods. Examples include carob bean gum, guar gum, and lecithin, thickening agents often used to give ice cream its rich texture.

Coloring Agents Coloring agents are used to improve the appearance of some foods as well as many drugs and cosmetics. Examples include FD&C Red No. 40, an orange-red dye used in puddings, drinks, and gelatins; and tartrazine (FD&C Yellow No. 5), a dye used in many drinks, cereals, preserves, and ice creams.

RISK FACTORS
▶ ▶ ▶ ▶ ▶ ▶

The use of additives in foods and beverages is controversial. Certain additives, most notably MSG and the coloring agent tartrazine, seem to trigger physical reactions such as hives in people with sensitivities or allergies to these chemicals. The role of additives in causing certain kinds of cancers is also the subject of debate and research.

Given these problems, some consumers argue that additives should not be used. Most food additives, however, serve necessary functions. They make foods safer, tastier, and more nutritious. In the case of preservatives, the risk of bacterial contamination outweighs any health risks from the chemical preservative. Food coloring, however, may be less necessary because these agents are usually added for purely cosmetic reasons.

The FDA attempts to minimize the risks of food additives by requiring thorough testing of any new additives and periodically reviewing additives that have already been approved. Unless you know that you are allergic to a particular food additive, you do not need to be overly concerned about the effects of additives in the food you eat. If you are subject to allergies, however, it is important to know the ingredients of the foods you eat and to avoid those additives that cause physical reactions. (See also FOOD ALLERGIES AND INTOLERANCES; FOOD LABELING; FOOD PRESERVATION METHODS; FOOD SAFETY; ORGANIC FOOD; FOOD AND DRUG ADMINISTRATION, 7.)

▶ FOOD ALLERGIES AND INTOLERANCES

Food allergies are abnormal immunologic reactions to food. A food allergy occurs when the body reacts to the protein in a specific food by producing *histamines.* These chemicals irritate the body tissues, producing a range of symptoms, some of which are potentially life-threatening.

Food intolerances are not the same as food allergies, although the two sometimes have similar symptoms. Food intolerances are abnormal reactions that generally do not involve the immune system. Instead, food intolerances typically result from the body's inability to digest or tolerate certain foods or FOOD ADDITIVES because of a lack of particular enzymes (chemicals that speed up certain processes in the body). For example, many people have a *lactose intolerance,* the inability to digest the natural sugar in milk, because they don't have enough of the enzyme *lactase.*

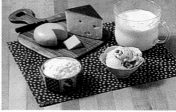

Food Allergy. *Sensitivity to cows' milk is a common food allergy, especially in young children.*

Symptoms of Food Allergies and Intolerances In most cases, the symptoms of food allergies and intolerances are simply unpleasant. They may include one or more of the following: abdominal pain, nausea, vomiting, diarrhea, hives, eczema, faintness, nasal congestion, sneezing, and swelling of the lips, tongue, throat, eyes, and face.

CONSULT A
PHYSICIAN

The most severe form of allergic reaction to food is *anaphylactic shock,* a sudden severe drop in blood pressure and collapse of the cardiovascular system. Anaphylactic shock requires emergency medical treatment.

Common Food Allergies   Foods that most often trigger allergic reactions include milk, eggs, soybeans, shellfish, wheat, and nuts. A few food additives also trigger allergies in some individuals. Many young children develop food allergies, but they often outgrow them by age 6. Adults with food allergies usually suffer from other allergic conditions, such as asthma or hay fever.

Identifying Food Allergies   Some food allergies cause an immediate reaction that makes them easy to identify. However, other foods can take hours or days to cause a reaction and are therefore not easy to pinpoint. Physicians diagnose these food allergies by taking an extensive personal history and by performing a variety of tests. If a specific food allergy cannot be identified, a physician may prescribe antihistamines or other drugs to relieve the symptoms. (See also ANTIHISTAMINES AND DECONGESTANTS, 7.)

Many people believe they have food allergies when, in fact, food intolerance or some other problem is responsible for their discomfort. For example, emotional and physical stress can interfere greatly with the digestion of food, causing symptoms similar to those produced by food allergies and intolerances. Consulting a physician and a dietitian can help determine whether particular symptoms are caused by a food allergy, a food intolerance, or some other problem.

Managing Reactions to Food   The only way to prevent abnormal reactions to food is to avoid the foods that trigger such reactions. People who must restrict their DIETS because of food allergies or intolerances should make sure that they are still eating a balanced diet. (See also ALLERGIES, 3.)

▶ FOODBORNE ILLNESS

Foodborne illnesses are illnesses caused by eating contaminated food. Food can be contaminated by a variety of microorganisms, including bacteria, viruses, parasites, and toxins. Symptoms of foodborne illnesses include loss of appetite, abdominal pain, nausea, vomiting, and diarrhea. Symptoms usually pass within a few hours, but some foodborne illnesses can be severe or even fatal.

Bacterial Foodborne Illnesses   Most foodborne illnesses (an estimated 8 million each year in the United States) are caused by bacteria. *Staphylococcus aureus* bacteria can spread if a food handler sneezes or coughs on food or if food preparers have open wounds on their hands. Gastrointestinal symptoms of "staph" infection appear within 1 to 6 hours after the food is eaten. *Clostridium perfringens* bacteria may contaminate cooked meat that is allowed to stand for several hours at room temperature. Symptoms such as diarrhea and abdominal pain appear 8 to 22 hours after the food is eaten. *Salmonella* bacteria, which cause millions of cases of foodborne illness each year, can be life-threatening to infants and elderly people. About 12 to 48 hours after a person eats food contaminated with salmonella, typical symptoms of foodborne illness appear and may be accompanied by

RISK FACTORS
▶ ▶ ▶ ▶ ▶ ▶

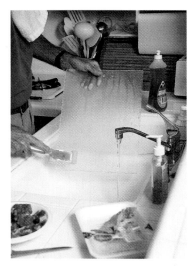

Foodborne Illness. *To prevent foodborne illness, a cutting board should be washed thoroughly in warm soapy water after use, especially when it has come into contact with raw meats.*

fever. Salmonella are often found in poultry, eggs, and meat. Cooking these foods thoroughly destroys these bacteria. *Campylobacter jejuni* may contaminate raw and undercooked meat and poultry, untreated water, and milk that has not been pasteurized. Like salmonella, these bacteria can be destroyed by thorough cooking. Symptoms, which appear 1 to 7 hours after infection, include diarrhea, abdominal pain, and cramps.

Botulism is a rare but very dangerous type of foodborne illness. It occurs when bacteria multiply in sealed containers of food that have been processed at too low a temperature. The bacteria that cause botulism (*Clostridium botulinum*) produce a *toxin* that cannot be destroyed by heating the food. If a can is swollen or leaking, or if the safety button on a jar lid has popped up, the container may be contaminated and should be returned to its place of purchase. Symptoms of botulism include muscle paralysis and double vision in addition to the more typical symptoms of foodborne illness. The condition is potentially fatal and must be treated immediately by a physician.

Traveler's diarrhea is caused most often by drinking water or eating foods contaminated with the common intestinal bacterium *Escherichia coli*. E. coli causes severe diarrhea that can last several days. When traveling abroad, avoid untreated water, uncooked milk products, salads, and raw fruits and vegetables that you cannot peel, unless you are sure that they are safe.

One strain of E. coli bacteria has particularly severe effects and can even cause death. These bacteria may contaminate raw or undercooked ground beef, unpasteurized milk, and produce. To be safe, hamburger meat should be well cooked, so that the meat inside reaches a temperature of at least 160°F (71°C).

Listeria monocytogenes can cause *listeriosis,* a serious disease that poses a particular risk to pregnant women, infants, and people who have weakened immune systems. These bacteria may contaminate poultry and seafood, eggs, raw and undercooked meat, produce, and improperly processed dairy products. *Shigellosis* is an intestinal infection caused by Shigella bacteria. These bacteria are found in foods that have been contaminated by the feces of an infected person.

Other Sources of Foodborne Illnesses Contaminated or spoiled seafood can transmit various foodborne illnesses. For example, the *hepatitis* virus can be spread by raw shellfish from waters contaminated with sewage.

RISK FACTORS ▶ ▶ ▶ ▶ ▶ ▶

Foodborne illness may also result from eating foods contaminated by *parasites*. Trichinosis, for example, is caused by a foodborne parasite. The *Cyclospora cayetanesis* parasite made thousands of people ill in 1996 and 1997 after they ate contaminated raspberries imported from Guatemala. *Toxoplasmosis,* a disease that can affect the central nervous system, is transmitted by a parasite that is sometimes found in pork and other meat. Some parasites, such as those in the genus *Cryptosporidium,* may enter the water supply and cause illness (See also TRICHINOSIS, **2.**)

Certain foods, including peanuts, potatoes, and some wild mushrooms, can themselves produce toxins that can cause illness. Occasionally, *insecticide* or *pesticide* residue on foods can create symptoms of foodborne illness.

Prevention   In most cases, foodborne illnesses are the result of unsafe food-handling practices. Many cases of foodborne illness can be prevented by following basic FOOD SAFETY guidelines: Clean all food preparation areas with hot, soapy water; cook foods at temperatures high enough to kill bacteria; and cool and refrigerate foods promptly. (See also BACTERIAL INFECTIONS, **2**; DIARRHEA, **2**; PARASITIC INFECTIONS, **2**; SALMONELLA INFECTIONS, **2**; VIRAL INFECTIONS, **2**; VOMITING, **2**.)

HEALTHY CHOICES

▶ FOOD CRAVING

A food craving is a strong desire to eat a certain food. While researchers are not quite sure why food cravings occur, many believe that they are caused by both physiological and psychological factors. Whatever their sources, food cravings are sometimes powerful enough to produce episodes of compulsive overeating in some people.

Physiological Cravings   A physiological craving reflects a physical need for a food. A craving for foods high in CARBOHYDRATES has been noted in people who exercise heavily, for example. This craving may come from the lowered blood sugar levels resulting from exercise, a condition best remedied by carbohydrate consumption. Some cravings seem to be associated with natural bodily rhythms, such as the menstrual cycle. For example, some women crave carbohydrate foods after they ovulate; they may eat as many as 500 extra calories a day just before menstruation. These extra calories may be needed to make the uterus ready for pregnancy. Cravings for salty foods during pregnancy are also common and are explained by the body's increased need for SODIUM during pregnancy. Other cravings may have evolved to protect the human species. Many people tend to eat foods higher in fat during the fall and winter months. This increased calorie intake may result from the historical necessity for human beings to stay warm in cold weather; it was probably a great survival benefit when people faced long periods of exposure to cold. Most Americans now spend most of the cold months in warmly heated buildings, but they may still experience such cravings.

Psychological Cravings   A psychological craving is a strong desire for a particular food in the absence of a physical need for the food. The sources

Psychological Cravings. *Some cravings are extremely strong and can be made worse by a rigid, strict diet.*

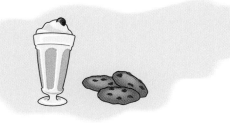
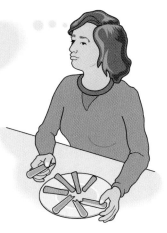

of psychological cravings for specific foods are not well understood. Most likely, they result from associations, conscious or subconscious, of foods with pleasant experiences or sensations in a person's past. For example, the feelings of comfort provided by foods such as ice cream or cookies that were given as rewards during childhood could explain cravings for those foods. A strict diet may also result in psychological cravings.

HEALTHY CHOICES

Coping with Food Craving Many nutrition experts think that understanding the basis of food cravings can help people keep them under control. Moderation in eating desired foods, rather than total denial, is recommended to avoid cravings that can result in overeating. (See also APPETITE; WEIGHT MANAGEMENT.)

▶ FOOD ENERGY   see ENERGY, FOOD

▶ FOOD GUIDE PYRAMID
The Food Guide Pyramid is a recommended method of planning a BALANCED DIET. It divides foods into categories according to the kinds of NUTRIENTS they supply, using a pyramid-shaped diagram to indicate the quantities that should be consumed daily from each group. The pyramid is a useful tool for understanding nutrition because it shows visually how much each food group contributes to a balanced diet. It reminds people at a glance which foods to focus on, which to eat sparingly, and how to balance the types of foods to maintain good health.

How the Pyramid Works The Food Guide Pyramid was developed by the U.S. Department of Agriculture (USDA). It organizes foods into five

Food Guide Pyramid. *The USDA's Food Guide Pyramid is an excellent tool for planning a balanced diet.*

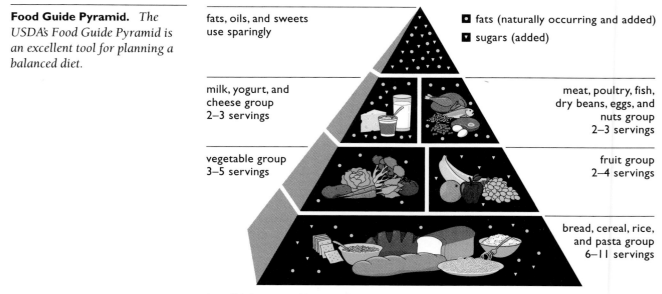

fats, oils, and sweets
use sparingly

◨ fats (naturally occurring and added)
◪ sugars (added)

milk, yogurt, and
cheese group
2–3 servings

meat, poultry, fish,
dry beans, eggs, and
nuts group
2–3 servings

vegetable group
3–5 servings

fruit group
2–4 servings

bread, cereal, rice,
and pasta group
6–11 servings

Source: U.S. Department of Agriculture/U.S. Department of Health and Human Services.

groups, with an additional sixth category (see illustration: Food Guide Pyramid). All are arranged in a four-tiered triangle that illustrates the relative quantities to be consumed from each group. The group at the pyramid's broad base (the BREAD, CEREAL, RICE, AND PASTA GROUP) is recommended as the largest source of CALORIES in the diet. FATS, OILS, AND SWEETS (a category of foods this is not one of the five basic food groups) is placed at the narrow top of the pyramid, indicating that these foods should be consumed in small quantities. Food groups on the lower levels of the pyramid make up the bulk of a healthy diet. Foods in the middle of the pyramid should be eaten in moderate amounts.

Using the System   The pyramid diagram indicates how many servings of each type of food should be consumed per day. For each food group, there is a range of recommended servings: for example, 3 to 5 servings daily from the VEGETABLE GROUP. Nutritional needs vary according to age and level of activity. Women and smaller people generally need less food than men and larger people. Older adults and women who are less active should eat a number of servings close to the low end of the range. Children, teenage girls, active women, and less active men should choose a number near the middle of the range, and active men and teenage boys need the maximum number of servings from each group.

To use the Food Guide Pyramid, you need to know the amount of food that makes up one serving. A single serving of meat, for example, is 3 ounces cooked, a portion about the size of a deck of cards. Because many people eat twice this amount in a single meal, they should be aware that in this case, they are actually consuming two servings of meat. Similarly, a serving of vegetables is about half a cup of cooked vegetables, a portion the size of a small person's fist. If you usually eat less than this amount, your serving of vegetables counts only as a partial serving. The DIETARY GUIDELINES published by the USDA offer a complete guide to the serving sizes recommended for the basic food groups.

HEALTHY CHOICES
●●●●●●●●●●●●

A healthful diet will include a variety of foods from each of the five basic food groups. Eating different foods each day will help you get all the nutrients your body needs. Some things you eat are combinations of foods from several different groups. Sandwiches, pizza, and lasagna are examples of such foods. To count these foods toward your daily number of servings, you should know what ingredients they contain and count each one as a serving (or partial serving) from the appropriate food group. (See also EXCHANGE SYSTEM; FRUIT GROUP; MEAT, POULTRY, FISH, DRY BEANS, EGGS, AND NUTS GROUP; MILK, YOGURT, AND CHEESE GROUP.)

▶ **FOOD LABELING**   Food labeling is the displaying of important information about a food product on the outside of its package. Food labels include the name of the product; the net contents or net weight of the package; and the name or location of the manufacturer, packer, or distributor. In addition, labels on processed, packaged foods must specify their ingredients and list nutritional information. Some food labels also include a freshness date.

List of Ingredients   Federal regulations require that labels for any food made with more than one ingredient must list the ingredients,

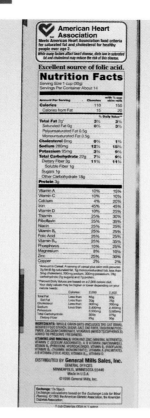

Food Label. *The first part of a nutrition label lists nutritional information based on one serving, including the number of calories and amounts of protein, carbohydrates, fat, and sodium. The second part lists the percentage of U.S. recommended dietary allowances for protein and seven essential vitamins and minerals.*

including certain FOOD ADDITIVES. The ingredients must be displayed in descending order based on weight. For example, if a breakfast cereal package lists its ingredients as "sugar, corn, salt, and malt flavoring," then the product contains more sugar (by weight) than any other single ingredient.

Nutrition Facts and Daily Values   The law requires nutrition labeling for almost all foods. Under the title "Nutrition Facts," a food label specifies serving size and provides detailed information about the amount of particular NUTRIENTS per serving. The label also shows the number of CALORIES per serving and indicates how many of these calories come from fat.

Labels display, by weight, the amount of FAT, CHOLESTEROL, SODIUM, CARBOHYDRATES, dietary FIBER, and PROTEIN in the food, as well as "% Daily Values." *Daily Values* percentages provide a general idea of how the amount of each nutrient supplied by one serving compares with the total nutritional needs of a person who consumes 2,000 calories daily. Food labels also include Daily Values for vitamins A and C, calcium, and iron. Thus, if a label says that one serving provides 25 percent of the Daily Value of vitamin C, that means that it provides one-fourth of a person's daily nutritional need based on a 2,000-calorie diet. Manufacturers may also voluntarily list additional nutrients on food labels. (See also RECOMMENDED DIETARY ALLOWANCE.)

People can use Daily Values as a reference to help them determine how particular food products may (or may not) fit into their daily diet. For example, people may increase their intake of foods high in certain vitamins or minerals that their diet may be lacking. Or, knowing that fat and cholesterol can increase their risk of heart disease, people can limit their intake of these substances to no more than 100 percent of the Daily Value.

Daily Values can also keep people from misinterpreting the meaning of nutrient weights. For example, 140 mg of sodium sounds like a large amount, but it actually represents less than 6 percent of the Daily Value for sodium. By comparison, 5 grams of saturated fat seems like a small amount. However, 5 grams represents 25 percent of the Daily Value of saturated fat.

Nutritional Claims   The government forbids manufacturers to make certain misleading nutritional claims on labels. In addition, federal law quantitatively defines the meaning of various terms. For example, a "low-calorie" food must contain no more than 40 calories per serving, while a "low-sodium" food must have 140 mg or less of sodium. A "low-fat" food must have no more than 3 grams of fat per serving, while a food that is "fat free" must contain less than 2 grams of fat. For a food to be labeled "high in" a particular nutrient, it must contain 20 percent or more of the Daily Value of that nutrient.

Health Claims   The government allows manufacturers to make certain claims on food packaging to link nutrients or foods with the risk of disease or health-related conditions. Claims that are allowed include links between calcium intake and lowered risk of osteoporosis; fat consumption and some cancers; and saturated fat and cholesterol intake and heart disease. However, federal regulations require that any such health claims must be supported by scientific evidence. The claims must also meet specific requirements in the way they are expressed.

Food Product Dating Food product dating, which is generally not required by law, indicates how long a product will remain fresh and wholesome. A packaged food may be labeled with a *sell by date* or a *pull date,* which is the last date on which the store should sell it. Foods such as meat and milk usually remain fresh for several days after the indicated date. A package may also have a *best-if-used-by date,* which is the last date on which a product should be used for optimal freshness.

Regulating Labeling The *Food and Drug Administration* (FDA) is the federal agency responsible for regulating food labeling. The FDA controls the use of information and claims on food labels. FDA regulations focus on the nutritional needs of average Americans. (See also DIETARY GUIDELINES; FOOD AND DRUG ADMINISTRATION, 7.)

· ·

▶ **FOOD PRESERVATION METHODS** Food preservation methods slow the spoiling of food. All foods eventually spoil, but preservation keeps food fresh so that it can be shipped long distances, eaten out of season, or stored for long periods in case of shortages. All of these factors reduce waste and help to ensure a steady food supply. In addition, food preservation prevents illnesses caused by bacteria and other microorganisms and increases the quality and variety of food that is available.

How Food Spoils *Enzymes* in fruits and vegetables cause them to ripen. Once they are ripe, however, the action of enzymes continues, and the food eventually spoils. *Microorganisms,* including molds, yeasts, and bacteria, cause changes in food that may give it an unpleasant taste or odor. They may also produce harmful substances in the food.

Many methods of food preservation have been developed over the years. Some have been around for centuries, while others use new technology. Food preservation methods include drying, pasteurization, canning, refrigeration, freezing, chemical preservation, and irradiation.

Methods Using Heat *Drying,* one of the oldest methods of food preservation, uses heat. Food can be dried in sunlight or by special machinery that circulates hot air. Both methods remove water from the food so that enzymes and microorganisms are destroyed. Fruits, beans, legumes, meat, fish, and milk are just a few of the many foods that can be dried. Dried foods may be eaten as they are or mixed with water to restore their original texture.

Pasteurization (a process invented by and named after French chemist Louis Pasteur) is used for liquids, such as milk and juice, to kill disease-causing bacteria and to extend shelf life. While pasteurization destroys disease-causing organisms, it does not kill all of the bacteria that cause spoilage. Therefore, although the liquid will stay fresh longer, it will spoil eventually. This is why even pasteurized milk is kept refrigerated. *Ultrapasteurization,* or *sterilization,* is a process in which foods are heated to even higher temperatures, destroying all microorganisms and preventing spoiling. Sealed, sterilized foods, such as milk, can be stored outside of the refrigerator until the package is opened.

Canning is another heating process that keeps food fresh. Foods are sealed in metal or glass containers before they are heated. Canned foods are usually as high in nutrients as fresh foods—sometimes more so, because they are usually canned at the peak of freshness, whereas fresh foods may be stored for several days and during that time may lose some of their nutritional value. Canned foods can be purchased at the store or prepared at home. Caution should be used with home-canned foods, as they can breed dangerous bacteria if they are not prepared properly. These foods should always be cooked thoroughly before they are eaten.

Methods Using Cold Low temperatures can also be used to preserve food. Many foods are shipped to markets in refrigerated ships, trucks, or trains. At the store, the food is kept in refrigerated cases. The temperature in *refrigerators* is just above freezing. The cold dramatically slows the growth of bacteria and molds in many foods, but does not stop it entirely.

Freezing is another low-temperature method of preserving food. Keeping food extremely cold greatly slows enzyme activity and the growth of microorganisms. Frozen foods will last a long time but not indefinitely. Like canning, freezing does not significantly affect the nutritional value of food.

Freeze-drying is a process that preserves food by first freezing and then dehydrating it. Frozen food is placed in a vacuum tank to remove the water, leaving a dry, spongelike solid. Freeze-dried foods keep their flavor and texture better than do foods preserved by drying. Instant coffee and soup mixes are sometimes prepared this way.

Chemical Preservation For centuries, people have added substances to food to preserve it. *Salt* can keep meat and fish from spoiling. *Sugar* is used as a preservative in jams and jellies. Ham and bacon are preserved, or *cured,* with a combination of salt and wood smoke. Vinegar, used in the *pickling* process, preserves pickles and other foods. Many FOOD ADDITIVES are used as preservatives in food processing as well as to improve taste and color.

Irradiation *Irradiating* food, or treating it with low levels of radiation, destroys microorganisms and insects. It also prevents new shoots from sprouting on potatoes and onions. When exposed to radiation, the food does not become radioactive. Irradiation can help to preserve many foods with little or no change in taste, texture, or nutritional value. The technology for irradiation is relatively new, and its use was approved for various foods by the U.S. Food and Drug Administration during the 1990s. Some people, however, remain concerned about possible health risks of irradiated foods. Under the new federal guidelines, certified ORGANIC FOOD cannot be processed in this manner.

One of the benefits of food preservation is that it reduces the risk of illness caused by spoiled food. But food preservation methods themselves may carry risks. Some scientists believe that not enough is known about certain food additives and irradiation. Researchers continue to study these and other food preservation methods to make sure that they are safe. (See also FOOD SAFETY; FOOD AND DRUG ADMINISTRATION, 7.)

► **FOOD SAFETY** Food safety means the principles and practices that keep foods free from the dangers of spoilage and contamination. For commercial food suppliers and public eating places, there are federal, state, and local

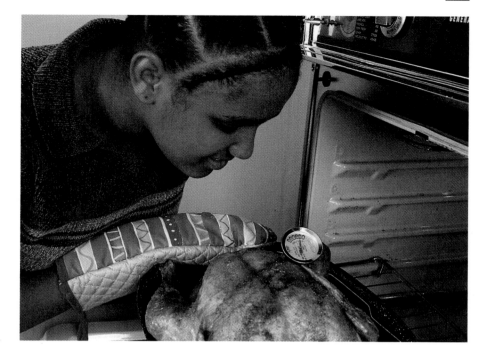

Using a Meat Thermometer.
It is important to cook meat thoroughly to prevent food poisoning. A meat thermometer should be used to tell when the meat is ready. For best results, insert the thermometer into the thickest part of the meat and make sure that it is not touching a bone.

health departments that regulate the storage, preparation, and serving of foods. These agencies conduct inspections to ensure food safety. By following the same principles at home, you can prevent FOODBORNE ILLNESSES, diseases that result from eating spoiled or contaminated food.

HEALTHY CHOICES
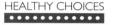

Keep Your Hands and Food Preparation Areas Clean   Cleanliness around food is very important in order to avoid *bacterial contamination.* Wash your hands with soap and water before and after handling food, after using the bathroom, after touching pets, and after blowing your nose or touching your mouth. Use a clean spoon to taste-test foods. Try to avoid preparing food if you are ill, and wear rubber gloves if you have an infected cut on your hand.

Wash utensils, cutting boards, dishes, and the sink with hot, soapy water. Use clean dishcloths and dish towels for every meal; wash sponges after each use and allow them to dry.

Prepare and Cook Foods Carefully   Many common foods normally carry bacteria. Always wash fruits and vegetables carefully to remove excess bacteria and pesticides that may be on the surface.

Meats, poultry, and fish require special handling. Do not allow these foods to thaw at room temperature. Instead, use a microwave oven, or thaw items in the refrigerator and then cook them immediately. Use a plastic rather than a wooden cutting board. Wash the board and knife in hot, soapy water, and rinse with very hot water. You may want to reserve a cutting board for meat, fish, and poultry only. If you marinate meat or poultry and want to serve the juices, boil them for several minutes first. Use a clean plate and utensil when serving the cooked food so that it will not be contaminated by its raw juices.

Use a meat thermometer when cooking poultry and pork (see illustration: Using a Meat Thermometer). Poultry should be cooked until the thermometer registers 180°F (82.2°C); pork should be cooked until the

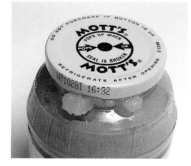

Signs of Contamination   *Do not use a container of food if it is bulging or leaking, or if the safety button has popped up.*

temperature reaches 160°F (71.1°C). Ground meat should also be cooked until its internal temperature is 160°F, or until it is no longer pink in the middle. When cooking any kind of meat, check the meat's juices. When the meat is thoroughly cooked, the juices will run clear. Fish is done when it is opaque and flakes easily.

Contamination of eggs with *Salmonella* bacteria is a growing concern. Discard cracked eggs, and cook eggs until they are firm, not runny, to destroy any bacteria. Also, avoid dishes that contain raw eggs, such as hollandaise sauce, homemade eggnog, and Caesar salad dressing.

When canning vegetables at home, follow reliable instructions, such as those provided by the U.S. Department of Agriculture.

Store Foods Correctly   Many foods are *perishable,* or liable to spoil. Use perishable foods quickly, and refrigerate or freeze leftovers immediately. The freezer must be kept at 0°F (−17.7°C), and the refrigerator temperature should be between 36° and 40°F (2.2° and 4.4°C) to maintain the safety of food. Allowing cooked food to sit at room temperature is dangerous. Harmful bacteria can grow at any temperature between 40° and 140°F (60°C), and they can take as little as 4 hours to multiply enough to cause foodborne illness. Turkey or chicken stuffing should be removed from the bird and refrigerated separately.

Store foods such as sugar, cereals, flour, and packaged mixes in containers with snugly fitting lids to avoid contamination by insects and rodents. Some whole-grain products (for example, wheat germ and whole-wheat flour) can spoil at room temperature. Refrigeration or freezing is necessary to keep them fresh.

Make refrigerator cleanup a regular task. Dispose of food that has been stored too long, especially if it has become moldy. Hard cheeses with mold are safe to eat, however, if you trim the mold away.

Purchase Foods with Care   When purchasing food, look closely at how well it is stored in the market. Do not buy foods that you find stored above the frostline in the supermarket freezer. If you are buying foods from a salad bar, make sure that the items are sufficiently chilled and protected from the coughs and sneezes of other customers. Buy fish from a reliable merchant who sells fresh fish and is knowledgeable about its sources. Never buy canned food if the cans are bulging or if the safety button on the lid has popped up. These are signs of *botulism* contamination, a dangerous type of foodborne illness. Do not use this food if you notice these signs at home. Instead, return it to its place of purchase (see illustration: Signs of Contamination). When you bag your groceries at the checkout counter, pack all cold foods together to keep them cold longer on the way home. Go directly home from the store when you have purchased perishable food, and put it in the refrigerator or freezer right away. (See also FOOD ADDITIVES; FOOD ALLERGIES AND INTOLERANCES; FOOD LABELING; BACTERIAL INFECTIONS, **2**; SALMONELLA INFECTIONS, **2**.)

▶ **FRUIT GROUP**   The fruit group is made up of plant foods such as apples, oranges, bananas, and melons. It is one of the five major food groups of the FOOD GUIDE PYRAMID. The fruit group is separate from the VEGETABLE GROUP

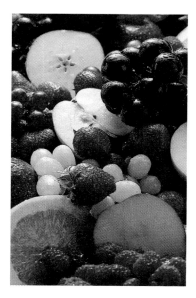

Fruit Group. *Fruits are rich in nutrients such as carbohydrates, vitamins, and minerals.*

HEALTHY CHOICES

because, although both fruits and vegetables are important sources of FIBER and many VITAMINS and MINERALS, fruits are high in a simple sugar called *fructose* and therefore are generally sweeter than vegetables.

Nutrition from Fruits   Most fruits are made up largely of CARBOHYDRATES (STARCH, SUGAR, and fiber) and WATER, with small amounts of PROTEIN and little or no FAT. They are fairly low in CALORIES. Different types of fruits are sources of different vitamins and minerals. For example, dark yellow and orange fruits, such as apricots and cantaloupes, are high in BETA CAROTENE and VITAMIN A. Citrus fruits, such as oranges and grapefruit, are excellent sources of VITAMIN C. Many fruits, including bananas, melons, cherries, and plums, are excellent sources of POTASSIUM.

Fruits are most nutritious when they are fresh, because they lose vitamin content if they are stored too long. Avoid peeling off edible skin such as that found on apples and pears; this skin often contains the richest concentration of nutrients and fiber. Fruits are also available frozen, canned, or dried. These processed fruits can be convenient when fresh fruit is not available. If you buy canned or frozen fruits, look for brands that do not have a lot of added sugar.

Daily Servings of Fruits   The Food Guide Pyramid recommends two to four servings of fruit each day. Ideally, at least one serving should be high in vitamin C. A serving is usually one piece of fresh fruit, half a cup of canned or cooked fruit, one-fourth cup of dried fruit, or 6 ounces (about 177 ml) of juice. Most Americans do not eat as many fruits and vegetables as nutritionists recommend. To add more fruits to your diet, try drinking fruit juice with meals, packing dried fruits as snacks, or sprinkling berries over breakfast cereal or yogurt. (See also BREAD, CEREAL, RICE, AND PASTA GROUP; DIETARY GUIDELINES; EXCHANGE SYSTEM; FATS, OILS, AND SWEETS; MEAT, POULTRY, DRY BEANS, EGGS, AND NUTS GROUP; MILK, YOGURT, AND CHEESE GROUP.)

GENETICALLY ENGINEERED FOOD   Genetically engineered food is food that has been changed through *biotechnology,* the scientific manipulation of biological organisms. Employing *genetic engineering* techniques, scientists can alter an organism's genetic material and improve plants, animals, and microorganisms used for food production. Genetic engineering is used to increase crop production, to reduce crop disease, and to produce better-tasting and more nutritious foods. Biotechnology includes familiar techniques, such as selective breeding and the creation of hybrids, as well new techniques involving the transfer of desirable genes from one plant to another.

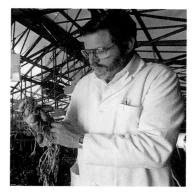

Genetically Engineered Food. *Foods can be genetically engineered to resist diseases and pests or to look or taste better.*

Benefits   Supporters of genetic engineering hope that it will lead to numerous and widespread benefits in food production. Some have already been achieved; many others are expected in the near future. For example, genetic engineering has led to the development of plants that are immune to certain destructive viruses. Scientists have developed potato and strawberry plants that are resistant to frost. Genetic engineering techniques have also been used to increase milk production in dairy cows. In the future, plants from which cooking oils are made may be modified to reduce their saturated fat content. Genetic engineering may also be used to make plants more resistant to insect damage, thus reducing the need for chemical spraying.

Controversies   Concern has been expressed, however, about genetically engineered food. Some people are disturbed by the idea of genetically modifying any organism, despite the fact that traditional agricultural methods have done this for hundreds of years. Environmentalists have expressed fear that genetically altered plants may drive out existing plant species or introduce new plant pests. Other concerns involve FOOD ALLERGIES AND INTOLERANCES. If, for example, a gene from a plant that is known to cause an allergic reaction (such as the peanut) is introduced into another plant, the altered plant may also cause an allergic reaction. For this reason, food labels must indicate that the allergen might be present in the new food. For all of these reasons, scientists are moving ahead cautiously with genetically engineered foods.(See also GENETIC ENGINEERING, 8.)

▶ GLUCOSE

Glucose is a carbohydrate that the body needs for energy. It is one of the basic fuels for all living cells. Although some foods contain small amounts of glucose, the body produces most of it from other CARBOHYDRATES such as STARCHES and other SUGARS. These are reduced to glucose by the digestive process.

Glucose's Function   Glucose has a simple chemical structure. It is absorbed directly into the bloodstream and carried to the cells. The cells then burn (or oxidize) the glucose to produce energy. Any unneeded glucose is converted to *glycogen* and stored in the liver and muscle tissues for later use. The glycogen can be released for conversion into glucose any time the body needs more energy. (See also LIVER, 1.)

Glucose.   *Glucose is a unit that makes up starches in fruits, vegetables, and grains. It is essential to body cells for energy.*

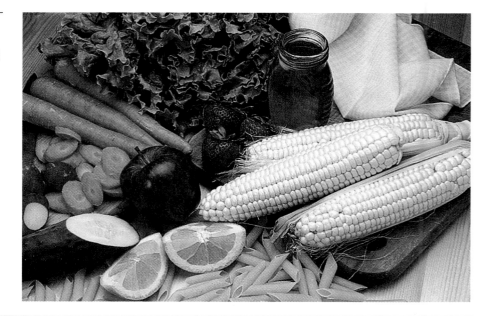

Blood Sugar Level   Regardless of the amount of carbohydrates a person consumes, the amount of glucose in the blood, or the *blood sugar level,* is usually kept within narrow limits. Several hormones help maintain these limits. For example, if the blood sugar level gets too high, the *pancreas* releases the hormone *insulin.* Insulin enables the cells to take in more glucose and thereby lower the blood sugar level. Conversely, when the blood sugar level is too low, the pancreas releases the hormone *glucagon.* Glucagon stimulates the conversion of glycogen in the liver into glucose, which is then released into the blood. This raises the blood sugar level. (See also PANCREAS, **1**; INSULIN, **7**.)

Blood Sugar Problems   Some people have problems with their blood sugar levels. For example, there may be too much sugar in the blood, a condition known as *hyperglycemia.* Symptoms include frequent urination, extreme thirst, and glucose in the urine. People who have chronic hyperglycemia have a disease known as diabetes. Most people who have diabetes do not produce enough insulin to take glucose from the blood. (See also DIABETES, **3**.)

Hypoglycemia is the reverse of hyperglycemia. People with hypoglycemia do not have enough sugar in their blood. Symptoms include hunger, weakness, sweating, and dizziness. People sometimes have minor, temporary attacks of hypoglycemia when they skip meals or eat meals that are too high in carbohydrates. Eating regular meals, snacking between meals, and eating a normal amount of carbohydrates usually alleviates the condition. A physician should be consulted if any of these symptoms persists for a long time. (See also BODY METABOLISM; DIGESTION; ENERGY, FOOD; ENERGY, PHYSICAL.)

CONSULT A PHYSICIAN

▶ # GRAINS   see BREAD, CEREAL, RICE, AND PASTA GROUP

▶ # HEALTH CLUB   see FITNESS CENTER

▶ # HEART RATE

Heart rate is the number of times the heart beats each minute. The rate increases during exercise and decreases while a person rests. Heart rate is largely an *involuntary* action, or one that a person cannot control. However, heart rate can be beneficially lowered by regular EXERCISE.

Heart rate can be measured by taking the pulse. Place the tips of your index and middle fingers along the line of the radial artery, on the thumb side of the wrist or in the front of the neck under the jaw (see illustration: Taking Your Pulse). Use a watch with a second hand to count the pulse for 10 seconds. Then multiply this count by 6 to calculate the total number of heartbeats per minute.

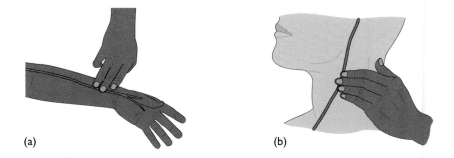

Taking Your Pulse. *Heart rate may be measured by taking the pulse at the (a) wrist or (b) neck.*

(a)

(b)

Resting, Maximum, and Target Heart Rates   The range for *resting heart rate* for an adult is between 40 and 80 beats per minute. People with a high level of *cardiovascular fitness* can pump more blood with each heartbeat; therefore, they tend to have heart rates on the low side of the normal range. People who are out of shape, however, typically have resting heart rates as high as 80 beats per minute or more. People whose fitness is poor when they begin an exercise program will see their resting heart rates drop, perhaps as much as 10 to 15 beats per minute.

The oxygen demands of intensive exercise require the heart to work harder and can greatly speed the heart rate. There are limits, however, to how fast the heart can beat. *Maximum heart rate* varies from person to person and gradually decreases with age. Maximum heart rate can be estimated by subtracting a person's age from 220. For example, a 20-year-old would have a maximum heart rate of 200 beats per minute (220−20=200).

Like all muscles, the heart grows stronger in response to significant levels of regular work. *Target heart rate* is a way of determining the amount of exercise necessary to increase cardiovascular ENDURANCE and achieve other health benefits of AEROBIC EXERCISE safely. This target rate is between 60 and 80 percent of maximum heart rate. For example, a 20-year-old person with a maximum heart rate of 200 will be exercising aerobically when the heart rate is between 120 (200 × 0.60) and 160 (200 × 0.80). A heart rate above 150 may indicate that a person who is just beginning an exercise program is exercising too vigorously. Below 120, the heart is not being required to work hard enough to achieve significant benefits.

HEALTHY CHOICES

■●●●●●●●●●●●●

For optimum results, you should do 20 to 30 minutes of aerobic exercise at your target heart rate. Because it is difficult to measure heart rate while exercising, you can also judge the intensity of your workout by your *rate of perceived exertion,* or how hard you feel you are working. On a scale of 0 to 10, where zero is no effort at all and 10 is maximum effort, try to maintain an effort level of 4 or 5: moderately strong to strong. Three to five sessions of such exercise per week can make a dramatic contribution to total health. You can also increase fitness by gradually increasing your exercise to longer periods at a faster pace. (See also FITNESS; FITNESS TRAINING; RUNNING; SPORTS AND FITNESS; HEART, 1.)

▶ **HUNGER**

Hunger is the unpleasant sensation of needing to eat. It is the body's way of saying that it is in need of fuel in the form of food.

Hunger should not be confused with APPETITE, which is a learned response to food and eating. Hunger has a purely physiological basis, although the exact mechanisms by which it is triggered are not well understood. Several theories have been suggested to explain how the body makes its need for fuel known to the brain. Factors may include the emptiness of the stomach, low levels of GLUCOSE or fat stores, and changes in hormone levels in response to food (or the lack of it).

However the message is communicated (it probably involves more than one signal), it is clear that the need for food is sensed in the section of the brain called the *hypothalamus*. The hypothalamus receives and processes many chemical messages from the body and issues a variety of appropriate "orders" in response. One of these is the order to eat, which the body senses as a physical need for food, or in other words, hunger.

In a similar way, the hypothalamus receives the message that the body has received enough fuel. It triggers the order to stop eating by producing the physiological sensation of fullness, or *satiety*. Simply put, hunger and satiety are sensations produced by the brain to act as "on" and "off" switches in regard to eating. (See also BODY METABOLISM; ENERGY, FOOD; HYPOTHALAMUS, **1**.)

▶ INTERVAL TRAINING

Interval training is EXERCISE that includes short periods of intense exertion (ANAEROBIC EXERCISE) alternating with periods of lower-level activity or rest. Interval training is an effective way to increase FITNESS because it gradually helps the body perform at higher levels of exertion for longer periods of time.

Exercising at maximum capacity soon leads to exhaustion. Interval training provides periods of rest or reduced activity after each burst of high-intensity activity. For example, a person might run vigorously for 3 minutes and then perform 2 to 3 minutes of gentle stretches, followed by 2 to 3 minutes of jumping jacks, followed by a couple of minutes of gentle jogging. The breaks in activity level enable the body to recover before going on to the next period of high-intensity effort. The training effect increases as the periods of high activity are lengthened and rest periods are shortened.

CONSULT A PHYSICIAN

Interval training is best for people who are already fairly fit and want to become more fit. People who are not used to exercising should check with a physician before beginning any exercise program.

▶ IRON

Iron is an essential MINERAL that plays a vital part in a variety of complex body processes. Although it is needed only in very small amounts, iron is one of the body's most important nutrients. It helps form *hemoglobin,* the oxygen-carrying component in red blood cells, and *myoglobin,* the oxygen-carrying component in muscle cells. Iron is also necessary for the manufacture of some of the body's most fundamental substances, including amino acids, hormones, and enzymes. The body normally obtains the iron it needs from foods. Liver, cereals, and leafy green vegetables are especially rich in iron.

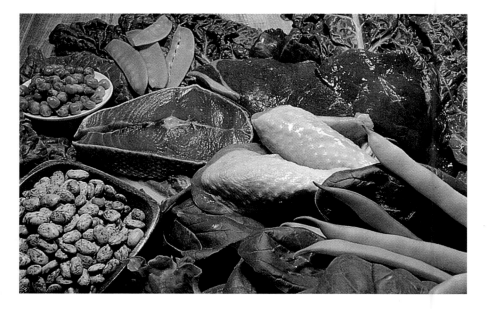

Sampling of Foods Rich in Iron. *There are two types of iron. Heme iron is found in meats, fish, and poultry. Nonheme iron is found in foods from plant sources, such as spinach, beans, and peas.*

Roughly 80 percent of the body's iron is contained in the hemoglobin in the blood. This iron is called *heme iron.* Foods of animal origin, such as meat and egg yolks, also contain heme iron. Foods from plant sources contain *nonheme iron,* which is not as easily absorbed by the body.

Iron Deficiency Even slightly depressed levels of iron in the body can interfere with the blood's ability to carry oxygen to cells, producing symptoms that include lowered energy levels and irritability. Greater iron deficiencies result in a decrease in the amount of hemoglobin in red blood cells, a condition known as *anemia.* Without enough hemoglobin, the blood cannot carry enough oxygen to the body's cells to support normal energy production. The resulting symptoms are fatigue, weakness, headaches, and reduced resistance to disease.

RISK FACTORS
▶ ▶ ▶ ▶ ▶ ▶

A diet low in iron, especially heme iron, can cause an iron deficiency because the body does not absorb enough nonheme iron. However, eating heme and nonheme iron together makes the body absorb the nonheme iron more effectively. VITAMIN C also improves the body's absorption of nonheme iron, if both are consumed at the same time. Drinking tea or coffee with meals, on the other hand, can interfere with the absorption of iron.

Any significant loss of blood can also produce a temporary iron deficiency. Although women lose only small amounts of blood during menstruation, they require more dietary iron than men do: 15 mg per day, as compared to 10 mg for men and 12 mg for boys between age 11 and 18. During pregnancy, however, a woman's iron requirement doubles. (See also RECOMMENDED DIETARY ALLOWANCES; MENSTRUATION, **6**; PREGNANCY, **6**.)

Iron deficiency is a significant health problem in the United States and even more so in developed countries where the average diet tends to be inadequate. In developed countries, between 10 and 20 percent of the population (mostly women) is estimated to have iron-deficiency anemia. The condition is treated by increasing the consumption of iron-rich foods and by taking iron supplements, often in conjunction with VITAMINS. (See also ANEMIA, **3**.)

▶ LIFESTYLE

Lifestyle refers to the way a person lives on a day-to-day basis. It includes attitudes, habits, and behavior. Your chosen lifestyle is a major influence on your health.

How Lifestyle Affects Health   Early in life, people develop certain *behavior patterns:* ways of acting alone and interacting with others. Those patterns involve decisions and trade-offs about work, social life, relationships, and many more elements of daily life that affect health. Behavior patterns and attitudes can have either a positive or a harmful effect on health. For example, people who eat a high-fat diet are increasing their risk of developing a number of serious diseases, including cancer and heart disease. On the other hand, people who eat a low-fat diet are reducing their risk of developing the same diseases.

HEALTHY CHOICES

One of the most significant behavior patterns that affects health is a person's activity level. In general, people who have an active lifestyle have more stamina, are sick less often, and live longer than people with a *sedentary,* or inactive, lifestyle. They tend to have a higher level of physical FITNESS and also have a more positive attitude about themselves. Some ways to lead an active life include having a job or a hobby, such as a sport, that involves physical exertion, or simply making time for EXERCISE in your regular daily schedule.

Several other lifestyle factors also are essential for promoting health and reducing risk. They include not smoking, eating a balanced DIET, drinking alcohol only in moderation, maintaining a recommended body weight, wearing seat belts in cars and helmets on bicycles, and getting enough REST. Attitudes can also affect health, however, in ways that are less well understood. *Stress,* for example, may be generally damaging to health and increase the risk of a number of unhealthy medical conditions. (See also ATTITUDES, **5**; STRESS, **5**.)

RISK FACTORS
▶ ▶ ▶ ▶ ▶ ▶

Making Healthful Choices   Although you cannot control every aspect of your health, you can make decisions about your lifestyle that have a

Lifestyle. *A healthful lifestyle is one in which people get regular aerobic exercise, eat and drink in moderation, eat a balanced diet, and do not smoke.*

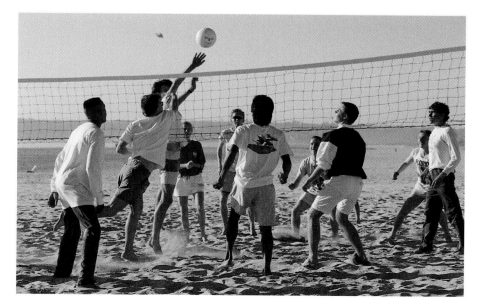

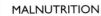
positive effect on your health and well-being. If you establish healthy behavior patterns early in life, you are more likely to maintain them as you grow older.

No two people will make the same lifestyle choices. The important thing is to establish the proper balance of diet, exercise, family, social life, work, and other factors in a way that is right for you. Finding behaviors and attitudes that are fulfilling will promote both health and happiness. (See also RISK FACTORS.)

MALNUTRITION

RISK FACTORS
▶ ▶ ▶ ▶ ▶ ▶

Malnutrition is an unhealthy condition caused by a lack of NUTRIENTS in the body. Worldwide, it is a major health problem responsible for millions of deaths each year. In the United States, severe malnutrition is much less common. However, marginal malnutrition, involving dangerously low levels of particular nutrients, affects many people in this country. Most such people are poor; others are on DIETS that do not provide their bodies with sufficient amounts of the right kinds of nutrients. Malnutrition may also result from diseases that prevent the body from absorbing or using nutrients properly.

Symptoms of malnutrition vary, depending on what nutrients are missing from the diet or which disease is the cause. In general, however, malnourished people experience diarrhea, weakness, weight loss, stunted growth, and susceptibility to infection. Children who are malnourished are often small for their ages and suffer from anemia and poor dental health.

Malnutrition Caused by Deficiencies in the Diet Dietary deficiencies may result when people have poor eating habits or limited food preferences, or when certain foods containing essential vitamins and minerals

Malnutrition. *In many less-developed parts of the world, malnutrition occurs as a result of social, economic, or geographic conditions such as floods, drought, poverty, war, disease, and ignorance.*

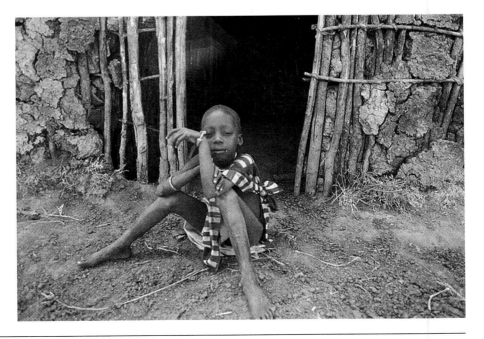

are unavailable. Common deficiencies include PROTEINS, CALORIES, VITA-MINS, and MINERALS. These deficiencies often overlap.

A person who does not consume adequate proteins and calories has *protein-calorie malnutrition*. This condition is the most common form of malnutrition among children in the developing world. Its primary symptom is stunted growth. Inadequate amounts of protein and too few calories can also produce a disease called *kwashiorkor* (kwah shee OR ker). Symptoms include a swollen face and stomach; patchy, flaking skin; weakness; stunted growth; and low resistance to illness. Kwashiorkor also damages vital organs such as the intestines, liver, and pancreas. This disease commonly affects children in poor countries after they stop getting nourishment from their mothers' BREAST MILK.

A deficiency of calories and nutrients leads to *marasmus,* another disease that is common in poor countries. A person with marasmus is very thin, with little or no fat under the skin. All muscles, including the heart, are wasted. This disease most commonly affects children 6 to 18 months of age. Since the brain grows rapidly at that time, marasmus often impairs brain development and learning ability.

Vitamin or mineral deficiencies may also cause malnutrition. The diseases that result vary, depending on the missing nutrient. For example, *anemia* is caused by a lack of iron or copper in the blood. (See also IRON; ANEMIA, **3.**)

Malnutrition Caused by Disease   Conditions and diseases that affect the body's ability to absorb or use the nutrients in food may cause malnutrition. Some of these conditions, such as tumors, infections, or inflammation, affect the intestines. Inadequate absorption may occur as a result of intolerance to *lactose* (a sugar in milk) or to a protein in wheat or rye flours, or as a result of a variety of rare acquired or inherited defects. The symptoms of intestinal problems usually include abdominal discomfort and weight loss.

Disturbances of the endocrine system or liver can also affect the body's use of nutrients. Diabetes mellitus is an example of an endocrine disease that can cause nutritional wasting. Finally, people with certain psychological disorders, including anorexia nervosa, may decrease their food intake to a level that causes malnutrition. (See also EATING DISORDERS; DIABETES, **3.**)

Groups Affected by Malnutrition   The group most seriously affected by malnutrition is children. The United Nations reports that 6 million children worldwide die as a result of malnutrition each year. Young children are particularly susceptible because they need more nutrients to fuel their growth and development. Poverty and lack of food, especially in developing countries, often prevent children from getting the nutrients they need. Even in the United States, an estimated 13 million children have trouble getting as much food as they need. Parental neglect and lack of nutritional knowledge often add to the problem.

The elderly are also prone to malnutrition. This problem may be the result of poverty or a lack of resources. It may also be a function of disability, social isolation, or loneliness, all of which tend to affect the elderly. A person who is lonely, for example, may have a depressed APPETITE and may lack the motivation to shop for food and prepare and eat healthy meals.

RISK FACTORS
▶ ▶ ▶ ▶ ▶ ▶

Alcoholics are also affected by malnutrition. Alcohol depresses the appetite so that many heavy drinkers eat poorly, if at all. Even heavy drinkers who eat well may be malnourished because alcohol prevents the absorption of nutrients, changes BODY METABOLISM, and increases the rate of excretion of many nutrients. (See also ALCOHOLISM, 7.)

Preventing Malnutrition Global malnutrition is a complex political and economic problem closely associated with poverty. It requires solutions that provide more effective food production and distribution systems, especially in developing countries. In the United States, social programs and agencies help ensure that many people in high-risk groups receive adequate nutrition. Still, many in need slip through these "safety nets" and suffer the damaging health effects of malnutrition. (See also NUTRITION; UNDERWEIGHT.)

▶ MEAT, POULTRY, FISH, DRY BEANS, EGGS, AND NUTS GROUP

The meat, poultry, fish, dry beans, eggs, and nuts group is a class of foods that includes beef, pork, poultry, fish, shellfish, eggs, nuts, beans, and peas. All of these foods are high in PROTEIN, which is an essential NUTRIENT for building new body cells. Many foods in this group are also important sources of VITAMINS and MINERALS. Some, however, are high in FATS and CHOLESTEROL, which have been linked to heart disease.

Foods in This Group *Meat* is the muscle or flesh of cattle (beef and veal), sheep (lamb), and pigs (pork, ham, and bacon). Meat is sold in cuts, such as "shoulder" or "loin," that indicate the part of the animal's body from which the cut was taken. *Organ meats,* such as heart, liver, and kidney, are especially rich in certain vitamins and minerals. *Processed meats,* including sausage, hot dogs, and luncheon meats, have been smoked or seasoned.

Poultry includes chickens, turkeys, ducks, geese, and game birds. Poultry is high in protein, rich in several important vitamins and minerals, and substantially lower in fat than meat. In addition to eating poultry, most Americans eat chickens' *eggs.* Eggs are a good protein substitute for meat, but egg yolks contain high amounts of fat and cholesterol.

Fish, another food in this group, may come from salt water (the ocean) or freshwater (lakes, rivers, and streams). Examples of saltwater fish are cod, halibut, tuna, and swordfish. Freshwater fish include trout and bass. *Shellfish* include shrimp, lobster, crab, and clams. Like poultry, fish is generally lower in fat and cholesterol than meat is.

Legumes are seeds that grow in a pod. They include *nuts* and *seeds,* which are plant kernels that usually come enclosed in a shell. Almonds, peanuts, pine nuts, and pumpkin seeds are examples of nuts and seeds. *Peas* and *beans,* including kidney beans, chickpeas, green peas, peanuts, and soybeans, are also legumes. As a class, legumes are lower in fat than are the other foods in this group. In addition, legumes (because they are plants) have no cholesterol. Legumes can also be eaten as part of the VEGETABLE GROUP.

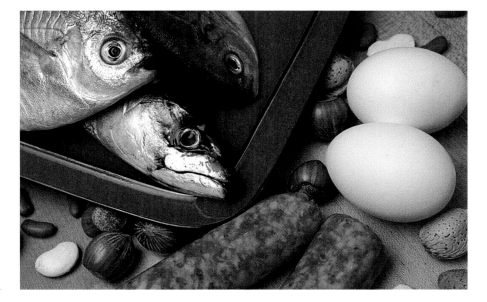

High-Protein Foods. *Foods in this group are high in protein and rich in many important vitamins and minerals.*

Nutrition from Meat, Poultry, Fish, Dry Beans, Eggs, and Nuts

Meat, poultry, eggs, and most fish provide complete proteins, whereas most nuts and legumes supply incomplete proteins. *Complete proteins* include all the *essential amino acids,* the components the body needs to build cells. *Incomplete proteins* lack one or more of these essential amino acids. Among plant foods, only soybeans, dried yeast, and wheat germ have complete proteins. However, you can easily obtain complete proteins by combining nuts or legumes with grains or meats. Together, these *complementary proteins* supply all the essential amino acids. For example, the beans and meat in chili con carne or the legumes and grains in a peanut butter sandwich complement each other to provide complete proteins. Complementary proteins need not be eaten at the same time to form complete proteins. As long as both legumes and grains are eaten as part of a balanced diet, the body will be able to combine the amino acids it needs to build and repair tissues.

Because excess protein cannot be stored in the body, it is a necessary part of the daily diet. Protein deficiency, although a major nutritional problem in some parts of the world, is rare in the United States. Nearly all Americans get the amount of protein they need for good nutrition, and many consume much more than they need.

In addition to protein, foods in the meat, poultry, fish, dry beans, eggs, and nuts group also provide significant amounts of VITAMIN A, VITAMIN B COMPLEX, and the minerals IRON, zinc, and phosphorus. Because exact nutrient content varies from one food to another, choosing a wide variety of foods from this group is the best way to ensure adequate amounts of these important nutrients.

Many foods in the meat, poultry, fish, dry beans, eggs, and nuts group are high in fat. Although fat is an important nutrient, most Americans eat too much of it. Overconsumption of fat, especially the saturated fat typically found in animal foods, can cause a person to become OVERWEIGHT and may lead to heart disease and other health problems. Nutritionists advise Americans to cut down on fat- and cholesterol-rich foods, particularly meat, and to eat more grains, fruits, and vegetables.

HEALTHY CHOICES
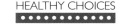

Daily Servings of Meat, Poultry, Fish, Dry Beans, Eggs, and Nuts
The FOOD GUIDE PYRAMID system recommends that people eat two to three servings of meat, poultry, fish, dry beans, eggs, or nuts per day. Sample servings are 2 to 3 ounces (57 to 85 grams) of cooked meat (a portion about the size of a deck of cards), one-half of a chicken breast, or a 3-ounce (85-gram) fish filet.

In general, you should usually choose foods from this group that are low in fat and cholesterol: poultry, fish, and legumes. Cooking methods also make a difference. When preparing poultry, for example, you should usually remove the skin, which contains a lot of fat. Avoid deep-frying foods or cooking them in large amounts of fat or oil. Lean cuts of meat should be chosen whenever possible. (See also BREAD, CEREAL, RICE, AND PASTA GROUP; DIETARY GUIDELINES; EXCHANGE SYSTEM; FATS, OILS, AND SWEETS; FRUIT GROUP; MILK, YOGURT, AND CHEESE GROUP; VEGETABLE GROUP; HEART DISEASE, **3**.)

▶ **MILK, YOGURT, AND CHEESE GROUP**   The milk, yogurt, and cheese group, sometimes referred to as the dairy group, is a class of foods that have milk as their main ingredient. Foods in this group include cheese, yogurt, and ice cream as well as milk. In the United States, most milk comes from cows; in many other countries, however, people also use the milk of goats, camels, sheep, and llamas. Milk and milk products are the chief source of calcium in the American diet, but this food group also provides many other NUTRIENTS.

Nutrition from Milk, Yogurt, and Cheese   Milk has been called the most nearly perfect food because it contains so many of the nutrients that the human body needs to live and grow. All milk products are rich in

Milk, Yogurt, and Cheese Group. *The foods in this group are good sources of calcium.*

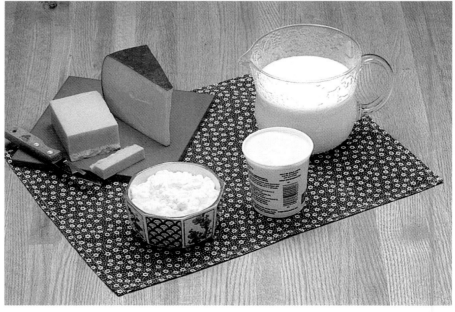

CALCIUM, a mineral essential to strong bones and teeth. Milk also contains a large amount of WATER as well as CARBOHYDRATES, PROTEINS, and FATS.

Milk also contains a variety of essential VITAMINS and MINERALS. It is a good source of vitamins A, E, and K, and riboflavin, a B vitamin. In the United States, VITAMIN D is added to milk because it helps the body use calcium. Besides calcium, milk contains minerals such as phosphorus, POTASSIUM, and SODIUM.

Because milk comes from animals, it is high in saturated fat and CHOLESTEROL, which have been linked to heart disease. Therefore, nutritionists recommend that people switch from whole milk to low-fat or skim milk and choose reduced-fat milk products.

Foods in This Group   Milk can be found in several forms. *Whole milk* is milk from which no fat has been removed, and *skim milk* is milk from which nearly all the fat has been removed. Milk is also available with only 1 percent (*low-fat*) or 2 percent (*reduced-fat*) fat by volume. These products are usually *pasteurized* (heated and cooled to kill disease-causing bacteria) and *homogenized* (blended to mix the fats into the liquid). Evaporated and condensed milk, from which much of the water has been removed, are available in cans. *Nonfat dry milk,* or powdered milk, is milk from which all liquid has been removed. Water is added to the powder to produce milk in liquid form.

The cream, or *butterfat,* in milk is used to make butter and ice cream. It is also sold separately as cream or half-and-half, a mixture of milk and cream. Butter is pasteurized cream that is stirred or churned until the fat particles form into a solid. (Because of its high fat content, butter is usually considered part of the FATS, OILS, AND SWEETS grouping of foods.) Ice cream is a frozen dessert made from cream or milk, sugar, and flavorings.

Yogurt, sour cream, and buttermilk are called *cultured milk products* because they are produced by adding cultures of harmless bacteria to milk or cream. This treatment gives them a thicker texture and a tangy taste. Special ingredients are also added to milk to make cheese. The ingredients cause the milk to separate into solid and liquid parts. The solids are then pressed into molds and aged to create cheese. There are more than 400 kinds of cheese.

People who are *lactose intolerant* have trouble digesting milk. They are missing or deficient in an enzyme (a chemical protein) necessary to break down *lactose* (milk sugar), the carbohydrate component of milk. An enzyme supplement is available to enable people who are lactose intolerant to drink milk. Special milk can also be purchased with the lactose in it already neutralized. Many people who are lactose intolerant find that they can eat cultured milk products and cheeses without experiencing problems.

Daily Servings of Milk, Yogurt, and Cheese   The FOOD GUIDE PYRAMID suggests two to three servings from this group per day. One serving equals 8 ounces of milk or yogurt or 1½ ounces of natural cheese. Teenagers and young adults, however, may need an extra serving to ensure that they get enough calcium. Pregnant and breast-feeding women may also need more milk and milk products. Low-fat and nonfat dairy products are healthy choices from this food group. (See also BREAD, CEREAL,

HEALTHY CHOICES
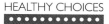

HEALTHY CHOICES
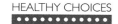

RICE, AND PASTA GROUP; DIETARY GUIDELINES; EXCHANGE SYSTEM; FRUIT GROUP; VEGETABLE GROUP; HEART DISEASE, **3**.)

▶ **MINERALS**

Minerals are inorganic nutritional substances that play a vital part in BODY METABOLISM, the complex life processes that occur within the body. There are many different minerals, each performing various functions. Some help in the movement of muscles, the transmission of nerve impulses, or the regulation of fluid levels in the body. Others are needed to form bones, teeth, and tissues or to regulate body temperature.

Minerals are classified into two groups, according to the quantities people need. *Macrominerals* are needed in relatively large quantities. This group of minerals includes CALCIUM, POTASSIUM, SODIUM, phosphorus, magnesium, and chloride (chlorine). *Microminerals,* also called *trace minerals,* are needed in smaller amounts. IRON, iodine, zinc, copper, manganese, fluoride (fluorine), chromium, selenium, and molybdenum are among the microminerals.

Deficiencies of most minerals are rare in the United States because most people get the amounts they need by eating a well-balanced diet. In addition, the body holds reserves of many minerals, releasing them as they are needed. Supplements of minerals such as iron and calcium are sometimes necessary, but these should be taken with a doctor's advice.

Nutritionists have compiled guidelines for the amounts of various minerals that should be consumed each day for good health.

The Food and Nutrition Board of the National Academy of Sciences is in the process of updating recommended intakes for minerals and VITAMINS. The chart of Recommended Dietary Allowances of Minerals lists those minerals that have not been updated (see chart: Recommended Dietary Allowances of Minerals). Calcium, phosphorus, magnesium, and fluoride were updated in 1997 and are shown in a separate chart (see chart: Dietary Reference Intakes [DRIs] for Four Minerals). Some of these amounts are now given as *adequate intakes,* or AIs. AIs are similar to Recommended Dietary Allowances (RDAs) and can be used as goals. There is not, however, enough scientific evidence to set a firm RDA for these nutrients. For four additional microminerals, suggestions are given as to estimated safe and adequate daily dietary intakes. The upper levels for intake of these elements should not be exceeded on a regular basis, since toxic levels may be only a few times the safe and adequate intakes (see chart: Estimated Safe and Adequate Daily Dietary Intakes of Four Trace Minerals).

Calcium Calcium is essential in building healthy bones and teeth. Deficiencies of calcium are relatively common and can contribute to *osteoporosis,* a disease characterized by a dangerous and sometimes crippling loss of bone mass. Calcium also helps muscles to contract, blood to clot, and nerves to send messages.

Potassium Potassium is essential to cell metabolism, the transmission of nerve impulses, and the functioning of muscles. Potassium also operates in conjunction with sodium to control blood pressure.

RISK FACTORS
▶ ▶ ▶ ▶ ▶ ▶

RECOMMENDED DIETARY ALLOWANCES OF MINERALS

Category (age, sex, or condition)	Iron (mg)	Zinc (mg)	Iodine (mcg)	Selenium (mcg)
Infants				
0–½	6	5	40	10
½–1	10	5	50	15
Children				
1–3	10	10	70	20
4–6	10	10	90	20
7–10	10	10	120	30
Males				
11–14	12	15	150	40
15–18	12	15	150	50
19–24	10	15	150	70
25–50	10	15	150	70
51+	10	15	150	70
Females				
11–14	15	12	150	45
15–18	15	12	150	50
19–24	15	12	150	55
25–50	15	12	150	55
51+	10	12	150	55
Pregnant females	30	15	175	65
Lactating females				
1st 6 months	15	19	200	75
2nd 6 months	15	16	200	75

Source: Reprinted with permission from *Recommended Dietary Allowances, 10th ed.* Copyright © 1989 by National Academy Press, Washington, D.C.

Sodium   Sodium fulfills many of the same roles as potassium, including the regulation of blood pressure. In people who are sodium sensitive, too much sodium in the diet (found in table salt and as an ingredient in most packaged foods) is associated with *hypertension* (high blood pressure), especially for salt-sensitive individuals.

Phosphorus   Most of the phosphorus in the body combines with calcium and forms calcium phosphate, which helps build and maintain bones and teeth. Phosphorus plays a variety of other roles in cellular metabolism, including helping with the transfer of *energy* and nutrients. Because phosphorus occurs in almost all foods, deficiencies are rare.

Magnesium   Magnesium performs numerous functions. It helps cells use energy, break down *proteins* and *carbohydrates,* transmit nerve impulses, and regulate body temperature. Magnesium deficiencies can be caused by persistent vomiting or diarrhea, kidney disease, diabetes, alcoholism, and the use of certain medications. Raw leafy green vegetables, nuts, whole-grain products, and seafood all are foods that are excellent sources of magnesium.

Chloride   Chloride performs several important functions. It helps maintain the acid-base balance in the digestive fluids of the stomach as well as in other body fluids. Chloride also helps transmit nerve impulses. Chloride deficiencies are rare, since most people get adequate amounts from table salt (sodium chloride).

Iron   Needed only in small amounts, iron performs a variety of important functions in the body. Most significantly, it is necessary for the formation of red blood cells. These blood cells transport oxygen to body cells, where the oxygen is used to produce energy. A deficiency of iron

DIETARY REFERENCE INTAKES (DRIS) FOR FOUR MINERALS

Age/Life-Stage	Calcium (mg)	Phosphorus (mg)	Magnesium (mg)	Fluoride (mg)
Infants				
0–5 months	210*	100*	30*	0.01*
6–11 months	270*	275*	75*	0.5*
Children				
1–3 years	500*	460	80	0.7*
4–8 years	800*	500	130	1*
Males				
9–13 years	1300*	1250	240	2*
14–18 years	1300*	1250	410	3*
19–30 years	1000*	700	400	4*
31–50 years	1000*	700	420	4*
51–70 years	1200*	700	420	4*
>70 years	1200*	700	420	4*
Females				
9–13 years	1300*	1250	240	2*
14–18 years	1300*	1250	360	3*
19–30 years	1000*	700	310	3*
31–50 years	1000*	700	320	3*
51–70 years	1200*	700	320	3*
>70 years	1200*	700	320	3*
Pregnancy				
≤18 years	1300*	1250	400	3*
19–30 years	1000*	700	350	3*
31–50 years	1000*	700	360	3*
Lactation				
≤18 years	1300*	1250	360	3*
19–30 years	1000*	700	310	3*
31–50 years	1000*	700	320	3*

*Note: This table presents Recommended Dietary Allowances (RDAs) and Adequate Intakes (AIs). AI values are followed by an asterisk.
Source: Reprinted with permission from *Dietary Reference Intakes* (prepublication versions). In press, National Academy Press. Courtesy of National Academy Press, Washington, D.C.

can result in *anemia,* a blood disorder that results in fatigue, weakness, and impaired mental ability.

Iodine Iodine occurs in the body in very small amounts. However, it plays a vital role in the activities of the *thyroid hormones,* which are involved in reproduction, growth, nerve and muscle function, and the production of new blood cells. Low levels of iodine can result in an enlarged thyroid gland, a condition known as *goiter.* On the other hand, too much iodine can also cause a condition resembling goiter. Iodine is normally added to table salt, so the average American will get enough in a normal diet.

Zinc Zinc performs a variety of functions in the muscles, skin, bones, eyes, liver, kidneys, and male reproductive organs. It helps to activate more than 70 different *enzymes* (substances that trigger body processes), increases the infection-fighting ability of white blood cells, and promotes the manufacture of sperm in men. It also plays an important part in growth and development. Zinc deficiencies sometimes occur and can inhibit growth and sexual maturation. Foods such as shellfish, meats, and whole-grain breads provide zinc.

Copper The micromineral copper interacts with iron to help prevent anemia. In addition, copper is involved in creating hair pigment, the sheaths surrounding nerve fibers, and elastin and collagen, elements of connective tissue. Copper deficiency is rare but can result from an inability to absorb it properly. Liver, shellfish, nuts, and mushrooms are among the many rich sources of copper.

Manganese Among its many important functions, manganese helps the body create fatty acids and cholesterol and metabolize carbohydrates. It is also necessary for normal bone and connective tissue development. Deficiency of manganese is unknown, but too much can cause serious problems such as weakness, muscle rigidity, and mental abnormalities.

ESTIMATED SAFE AND ADEQUATE DAILY DIETARY INTAKES OF FOUR TRACE MINERALS

Age	Copper (mg)	Manganese (mg)	Chromium (mcg)	Molybdenum (mcg)
Infants				
0–6 months	0.4–0.6	0.3–0.6	10–40	15–30
6–12 months	0.6–0.7	0.6–1.0	20–60	20–40
Children and Adolescents				
1–3 years	0.7–1.0	1.0–1.5	20–80	25–50
4–6 years	1.0–1.5	1.5–2.0	30–120	30–75
7–10 years	1.0–2.0	2.0–3.0	50–200	50–150
11+ years	1.5–2.5	2.0–5.0	50–200	75–250
Adults	1.5–3.0	2.0–5.0	50–200	75–250

Source: Reprinted with permission from *Recommended Dietary Allowances, 10th ed.* Copyright © 1989 by National Academy Press, Washington, D.C.

Manganese toxicity usually does not result from high dietary intake but from industrial contamination. Nuts, whole-grain cereals, dried beans, and tea are all rich in manganese.

Fluoride Fluoride is necessary to strong bones and teeth. It helps protect children's teeth from decay and may delay the progress of osteoporosis in adults. Fluoridated water, fish, and tea are dietary sources of fluoride. Fluoride can also be applied to the surfaces of teeth when they are brushed with fluoridated toothpaste.

Chromium The body needs chromium in order to make effective use of the sugar GLUCOSE, the primary food of cells. A deficiency of chromium in adults has been associated with diabetes. In children, it has been linked to slowed growth. Vegetables, whole grains, fruits, and cheese are high in chromium.

Selenium The micromineral selenium helps protect cells against damage from oxygen-derived compounds. A selenium deficiency is linked to heart problems and possibly to certain types of cancer. Foods grown in regions with selenium-poor soil may be low in this mineral. Too much selenium is also dangerous and can cause loss of hair and nails, damage to skin and teeth, and problems with the nervous system.

Molybdenum Molybdenum helps the body produce uric acid and use iron stored in the liver. It may also help prevent tooth decay. Deficiencies of molybdenum are unknown. Too much of this mineral can result in goutlike symptoms such as pain and swelling in joints. Peas, beans, and meats are the best sources of this trace mineral. (See also NUTRIENTS; RECOMMENDED DIETARY ALLOWANCE; VITAMINS.)

▶ **NATURAL FOOD** see ORGANIC FOOD

▶ **NUTRIENTS**

Nutrients are substances in food that are essential to good health. They build, maintain, and repair body tissues; regulate body processes; and provide fuel for energy. There are six essential nutrients of two basic types. The *macronutrients,* so called because they are required in large quantities, are carbohydrates, fats, proteins, and water. Minerals and vitamins, on the other hand, are needed only in very small amounts and are therefore classified as *micronutrients*. It is important to eat a varied and balanced diet because nutrients work together to maintain health (see chart: Basic Nutrients in Selected Foods).

Macronutrients CARBOHYDRATES provide energy in two basic forms: STARCH and SUGAR. A third type of carbohydrate, FIBER, is not digested but helps the body eliminate solid wastes by providing bulk, or roughage. Carbohydrates are found in large amounts in grains, vegetables, and

BASIC NUTRIENTS IN SELECTED FOODS

Food	Macronutrients			Vitamins			Minerals		
	Fat (g)	Protein (g)	Carbohy-drates (g)	Vitamin A (retinol equivalents)	Thiamine (mg)	Vitamin C (mg)	Calcium (mg)	Iron (mg)	Sodium (mg)
Apple (1 large)	1	—	32	11	0.04	12	15	0.4	—
Orange (1 large)	—	2	22	39	0.16	98	74	0.2	—
Bagel	1	7	38	—	0.12	—	13	1	379
Cracked-wheat bread (1 slice)	1	2	12	—	0.09	—	11	0.7	135
Kellogg's Raisin Bran (1 cup)	1	6	47	250	0.43	—	35	5	354
Broccoli, raw (½ cup)	—	1	2	68	0.03	41	21	0.4	12
Carrot, raw (1 medium)	—	1	6	1716	0.06	6	17	0.3	21
Reduced-fat milk (2%) (1 cup)	5	8	12	139	0.09	2	297	0.1	122
Skim milk (1 cup)	—	8	12	149	0.08	2	302	0.1	126
Tuna, in water (6 oz)	5	41	—	10	—	—	24	1.7	648
Ground beef patty, broiled (3 oz)	13	24	—	—	0.06	—	8	2.4	70
Bean and Cheese Burrito (2 pieces)	12	15	55	238	0.2	2	214	2.3	1166
Chicken, roasted (5.1 oz)	11	42	—	23	0.1	—	22	1.8	126

Source: U.S. Department of Agriculture, 1988. *Nutrient Database for Standard Reference.*

fruits. FATS are the body's source of reserve energy. They also insulate the body against excessive heat loss and help it to store and use vitamins. Foods high in fats include butter, meats, salad dressings, cheeses, and milk. PROTEINS build and maintain body tissues. Animal products (meats, poultry, fish, milk, and eggs) are high-protein foods. Vegetables, fruits, and grains also contain protein, but most of these proteins are incomplete. WATER is needed in large quantities to help digest food, carry other nutrients to cells, eliminate wastes from the body, and cool the skin.

Micronutrients MINERALS help maintain vital body processes, including the function of muscles, the manufacture of red blood cells, the transmission of nerve impulses, and the formation and maintenance of bones and teeth. VITAMINS help regulate numerous body processes. Both minerals and vitamins can be found in many types of foods.

▷ NUTRITION

Nutrition is the relationship between food and human health. Nutrition is also the scientific study of NUTRIENTS and the processes by which they nourish the human body.

Good Nutrition Versus Poor Nutrition   Good nutrition is vital to health and well-being. A varied, well-balanced diet, appropriate in amount, is the basic source of good nutrition.

Too little food, especially if much of it is low-nutrient food, results in MALNUTRITION, which contributes to many diseases and disorders. Too much food and too little exercise cause *obesity* and its associated medical problems. Imbalances in the diet also result in poor nutrition. For example, heart disease and some types of cancer may occur when people eat too much fat. Too much salt in the diet can aggravate hypertension (high blood pressure) in salt-sensitive individuals. People who eat large amounts of sugar may have inadequate VITAMIN and MINERAL intake, which can lead to a variety of health problems.

The Science of Nutrition   Nutrition is a relatively young science. It was not recognized as a distinct area of study until 1934, but it has grown in importance since that time. Much has been learned about the links between diet and health. For example, 40 years ago, many people had not heard of CHOLESTEROL. Now, most people know that a diet high in saturated fat and cholesterol may result in blocked arteries and can contribute to heart disease.

The science of nutrition covers a broad range of issues and concerns. Nutritional scientists investigate how the essential nutrients affect growth, disease, and metabolism. *Nutritionists* address questions about what foods people should eat and how changes in diet affect people. They study how

Good Nutrition. *Good nutrition starts with a well-balanced diet of healthful foods.*

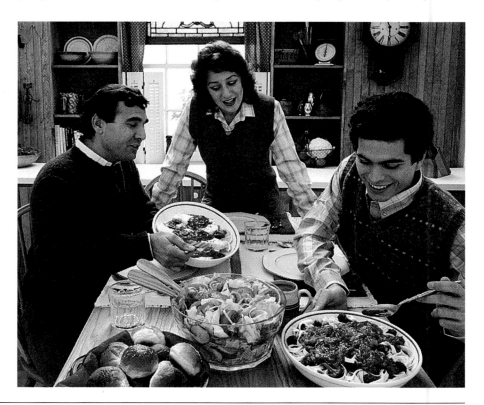

foods are digested, absorbed, and used by the human body. (See also BODY METABOLISM.)

Nutritionists also apply nutritional principles directly to the treatment of disease. *Nutritional therapy* adjusts diet to help cure or control diseases. For instance, many people with diabetes mellitus are able to control the disease without medication by regulating the amount of CARBOHYDRATES in their diet. In addition, a low-protein diet can slow the progression of chronic liver failure, and vitamin therapy is useful in treating certain kinds of cancer.

Dietetics Dietetics is the science of applying the principles of nutrition to the DIETS of individuals and groups. *Registered dietitians* are people who are trained to use those principles to plan diets. For example, dietitians develop low-fat diets for people who want to control blood cholesterol levels and lose weight; they design low-salt diets for people with hypertension. They also give people advice on shopping for foods and on making healthful choices in restaurants. (See also PHYTOCHEMICALS; CANCER, 3; DIABETES, 3; HEART DISEASE, 3; HYPERTENSION, 3; NUTRITIONIST, 9.)

▶ **ORGANIC FOOD**   Organic food, more accurately called organically grown food, is produced without the use of synthetic chemicals. No *chemical fertilizers, pesticides,* or FOOD ADDITIVES are used intentionally in producing organically grown foods.

Many people believe that organic food is more healthful than other food because organic matter, such as manure and compost (rotted leaves and other vegetable materials) are used as fertilizer instead of factory-produced chemicals. Some organic foods do contain less of such chemicals than do other foods. However, many organic foods contain some of the same chemicals as foods that are grown with chemical fertilizers and pesticides. They may be grown in soils that were previously treated with AGRICULTURAL CHEMICALS. The chemicals remain in the soil for years and affect crops that are grown there. In addition, if nearby farmers spray their crops with pesticides, the wind, rain, and groundwater can carry those chemicals to the fields of organic farmers.

Organic food contains essentially the same NUTRIENTS as other food. Organic food may, however, have retained more nutrients at the time of purchase than conventionally grown food. This may happen because organic food does not stay fresh as long as conventionally grown food; therefore, the food may not be kept as long in grocery store bins. Organically grown fruits and vegetables may be less attractive than other food, however, because pesticides are not used to keep insects from biting or boring holes in the skins. Organic foods are usually more expensive than other foods. Some of the additional expense comes from labor costs. Because no chemical pesticides or weed killers are used, weeds and insects must be removed by hand.

People who prefer organic food question the long-term safety of consuming agricultural chemicals. In fact, a few pesticides have been withdrawn from the market after decades of use because they proved to be potentially unsafe for consumption. In addition, organic food production

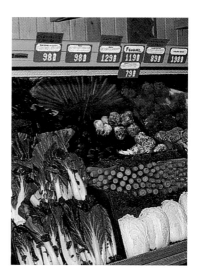

Organic Food. *Many supermarkets have set aside sections for organic foods.*

methods are generally thought to be less harmful to the environment, a concern of many consumers.

When you buy food, carefully compare the cost, appearance, and nutritional value of organic food to that of other food. In the 1990s, the U. S. government set out to establish standards for organic foods, including a definition of the term *organic*. The goal is to require that foods sold as "organically grown" or "organically produced," including produce, meats, dairy products, bakery products, and processed foods be certified by the U.S. Department of Agriculture (USDA). Among the proposed regulations are the requirement that at least 50 percent of the ingredients in a food labeled "organically produced" must be produced organically. Also, processed organic foods are not supposed to contain any nitrates, nitrites, or sulfites. (See also FOOD SAFETY; FOOD AND DRUG ADMINISTRATION, 7; AGRICULTURAL POLLUTION,8.)

▶ OVERWEIGHT

A person who is overweight is one who has an unhealthy amount of excess BODY FAT. This may be determined initially by measuring BODY MASS INDEX, or BMI. However, BMI can be misleading because it depends only on a person's height and weight; it does not measure the percentage of body fat. Because a heavily muscled body will weigh more than a slender one, a person with a high BMI may still be healthy. It is therefore common to check a person's waist measurement as well. A waist measurement of 40 inches for men or 35 inches for women, combined with a BMI of 25 or higher, means that a person is overweight. A person whose BMI is 30 or above is *obese:* overweight enough to be at a significantly higher risk of serious health problems. (See also WEIGHT ASSESSMENT.)

Excessive weight is a major health problem in the United States. More than half of American adults and approximately one-fourth of American children are overweight. This number has grown dramatically in recent years. Some experts claim that if the trend toward weight gain is not reversed, eventually nearly the entire U.S. population will be overweight. Others argue that the definition of overweight is inappropriate and overlooks other issues, such as eating habits and activity level, that have more influence on overall FITNESS. Most authorities agree, however, that people who are overweight have at least somewhat greater health risks than people who are not.

Causes Many factors can cause someone to become overweight or obese. Excess body fat builds up when the number of calories consumed exceeds the number expended. Calorie expenditure depends on an individual's BODY METABOLISM, the rate at which energy is used by the body. Some overweight people have very slow metabolic rates. In other cases, poor eating habits (especially a high-fat diet) and a lack of physical EXERCISE are the major causes of weight gain. The tendency to be overweight is to some degree hereditary. A person with an inclination to become overweight can easily gain weight over time if there is an increase in calories consumed or a decrease in calories burned. In many cases, hereditary and behavioral factors work together to cause excessive weight gain.

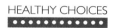

RISK FACTORS
▶ ▶ ▶ ▶ ▶ ▶

Health Risks Whatever the cause, being overweight or obese is bad for your health. It can increase your risk of high blood pressure, stroke, diabetes, heart disease, and certain types of cancer, for instance. The American Heart Association recently declared obesity to be a major risk factor for heart attacks. Extra weight can put strain on the back and on the joints of the hips and knees. Losing weight produces substantial health benefits for overweight and obese people. It improves general health, increases life expectancy, and often enhances a person's sense of well-being.

HEALTHY CHOICES
●●●●●●●●●●●●

Treatment The best way to lose excess body fat is to follow a sensible WEIGHT-LOSS STRATEGY that combines a reduction in calorie intake with regular, progressive physical exercise. To be safe, weight loss should be gradual: 1 to 2 pounds per week until the desired weight is achieved. FAD DIETS that involve a very low calorie intake do not produce good long-term results; lost weight is usually regained. Group weight-loss programs can offer information and support. Developing good eating and exercise habits will help keep the weight off once a goal is reached. (See also DIET AIDS; DIET FOOD; DIETS; RISK FACTORS; UNDERWEIGHT; WEIGHT MANAGEMENT.)

▶ PERSONAL TRAINER

A personal trainer is a person who is qualified to help an individual design and carry out an exercise program suited to his or her fitness goals and health concerns. A personal trainer may work at a FITNESS CENTER or visit private homes. The best-qualified trainers are certified by a reputable organization, such as the American College of Sports Medicine, the American Council on Exercise, or the National Academy of Sports Medicine.

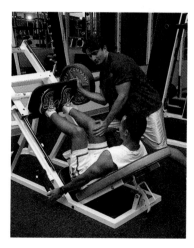

Personal Trainer. *A personal trainer can design an exercise program that meets your goals and fits your lifestyle.*

What Trainers Do Personal trainers help people begin and continue individualized exercise programs. Trainers instruct clients in the principles of exercise and guide them in the use of EXERCISE MACHINES and equipment. They may also provide nutritional information.

People hire a personal trainer for various reasons. They may want to improve their overall physical condition, or they may need help recovering from an injury or illness. Some people want a trainer to help them prepare for a particular sports event or activity. Others want a trainer first to help them learn to use unfamiliar equipment and then to assess their ongoing progress.

To create an individualized exercise program, a trainer considers the person's specific fitness goals and exercise preferences. The trainer also evaluates the person's current physical condition, including any health risks associated with lifestyle or family history.

▶ PHYTOCHEMICALS

Phytochemicals are chemical substances found in vegetables, herbs, and other plants. Most phytochemicals are not considered NUTRIENTS because they are not known to be essential to good health. However, many phytochemicals are believed to be beneficial to health. Researchers continue to find promising new classes of phytochemicals that can protect human cells from damage, inhibit processes that lead to cancer and other diseases, and possibly even retard the aging process. Phytochemical research is a relatively new field, however, and more studies are needed to establish a convincing connection between many of these chemical substances and their possible benefits.

To date, a number of studies have found potentially beneficial phytochemicals in a range of plants. Garlic and onions, for example, contain sulfur compounds that may partially detoxify cancer-causing agents. Broccoli and other related vegetables (for example, cauliflower, brussels sprouts, and cabbage) contain isothiocyanates, compounds that may discourage cancer by helping cell enzymes fight tumors. The peels of citrus fruits contain limonene, a chemical that may prevent breast cancer. Tofu, soy milk, and other foods made from soybeans are rich in isoflavones, substances that may inhibit cancer cell growth and division.

The notion of special disease-fighting or -preventing qualities in specific foods is nothing new. Since ancient times, folk medicine has promoted the benefits of certain foods and herbs and has developed tonics and treatments from plants. Contemporary research in cellular metabolism is beginning to explain why some of these substances work. Many foods recently identified as beneficial correspond closely to foods promoted in folk medicine. This has led some researchers to theorize that people's tastes may be partially shaped by an innate knowledge of what is good for them.

HEALTHY CHOICES
●●●●●●●●●●●●

The U.S. Department of Agriculture's Research Center on Aging is coordinating phytochemical research at universities around the country. The National Cancer Institute has conducted studies to examine how chemicals in common foods can fight cancer. Although more research needs to be done before the effects of phytochemicals on health are clear, studies have generally shown that eating a variety of fruits, vegetables, and whole grains is associated with a lower risk of cancer as well as other health benefits. Some experts predict that in the future, foods may be fortified with specific disease-preventing agents, just as today's foods are enhanced with VITAMINS and MINERALS. (See also BETA CAROTENE; BREAD, CEREAL, RICE, AND PASTA GROUP; FRUIT GROUP; VEGETABLE GROUP; VITAMIN B COMPLEX; VITAMIN C; VITAMIN E.)

▶ POTASSIUM

Potassium is an essential MINERAL that is present in all living cells. Along with SODIUM, it carries through the body the electrical charges that enable cells to function. Potassium helps maintain normal heart rhythm, the proper functioning of muscles, and the body's water balance. It also works to help the body regulate blood pressure. Although most foods contain potassium, the greatest quantities are found in vegetables (especially beans and potatoes), fruits (especially oranges and bananas), and whole grains.

Potassium Deficiency Because potassium is found in most foods, deficiencies are rare. However, they can occur with some digestive disorders

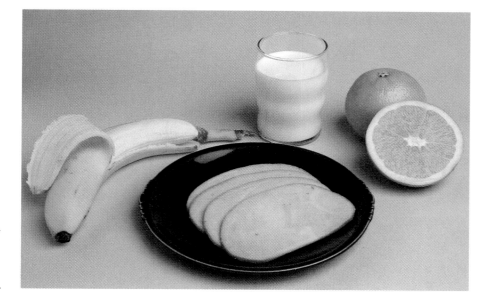

Sampling of Foods Rich in Potassium. *To maintain good health, a daily intake of at least 2,000 mg of potassium per day is suggested. Foods rich in this mineral include bananas, oranges, whole milk, and poultry and meats such as turkey and beef.*

and with continued diarrhea or vomiting, which results in the loss of potassium-rich fluids. Overconsumption of alcohol or aspirin as well as long-term treatment with certain other drugs, can also deplete the body's supply of potassium.

▶ PRESIDENT'S COUNCIL ON PHYSICAL FITNESS AND SPORTS

The President's Council on Physical Fitness and Sports was established in 1956 to encourage FITNESS and sports participation among all Americans. The council uses advertising, articles, special events, and awards programs to focus public awareness on the importance of staying physically active. It also encourages schools, business and industry, government, recreation agencies, and sports and youth organizations to develop and maintain physical fitness and sports programs for people of all ages.

One of the important goals of the council is to help young Americans achieve fitness. Among its major programs is the *President's Challenge,* which motivates and rewards students from age 6 to 17 to meet challenging levels of fitness in cardiovascular and muscular ENDURANCE, STRENGTH, FLEXIBILITY, and agility. (See also EXERCISE; FITNESS TRAINING; SPORTS AND FITNESS.)

▶ PROTEINS

Proteins are one of the four main groups of *macronutrients* (nutrients that the body needs in large amounts). Proteins are essential for the growth and repair of body tissues. Protein is a part of every cell and a key component in the structure of body tissues (such as hair, skin, muscles, tendons, and cartilage). Because protein is lost every day as cells wear out, it is essential to the daily diet.

The Composition of Proteins Proteins are made up of *amino acids,* chemicals that are referred to as the building blocks of the body. The body links the amino acids to form the proteins it needs.

Twenty-two amino acids build human proteins. Nine of them, called *essential amino acids,* must be supplied by food because the body cannot produce them. The body can manufacture the other 13 amino acids from other substances in food. Since amino acids cannot be stored in the body, it is important to get enough of them in your diet on a regular basis.

Dietary Sources of Protein Foods of animal origin, such as meat, poultry, fish, milk products, and eggs, supply *complete proteins* that include all nine essential amino acids. Although foods from plants, such as vegetables, seeds, grains, and nuts, also supply proteins, these usually lack one or more of the essential amino acids. They are therefore called *incomplete proteins.* You can get all of the essential amino acids from plant-based foods through *protein complementing:* eating a variety of foods throughout the day that, when combined, provide all of the essential amino acids. You may also rely on the few plant-based foods that provide complete proteins: soybeans, dried yeast, and wheat germ. (See also VEGETARIAN DIET.)

Many protein-rich foods from animal sources are high in FATS, and all lack FIBER. Therefore, you should try to get at least half of your daily protein requirements from plant sources. Good choices of animal protein sources are lean meat and fish, poultry without skin, and low-fat or non-fat milk, yogurt, and cheeses (see chart: Sources of Protein).

The Role of Proteins in the Body Proteins play an important and complex role in many body processes. As discussed earlier, proteins in food are broken down by DIGESTION into amino acids, which then combine to become new body proteins. The genes in each cell direct each person's body to manufacture a different assortment of proteins. In fact, the differences in the "codes" that each person's genes contain for making proteins cause the hereditary differences among people.

Proteins are either soluble or insoluble, and their role in the body depends on which type they are. *Insoluble proteins* (or fibrous proteins)

HEALTHY CHOICES
●○●○●○●○●○●○

HEALTHY CHOICES
●○●○●○●○●○●○

SOURCES OF PROTEIN	
Low-fat protein sources	**High-fat protein sources**
Most fish	Eggs (including the yolks)
Poultry without skin	Peanut butter
Lean meat	Most nuts and seeds
Low-fat or nonfat milk	Most cheeses
Buttermilk	Whole milk
Low-fat or nonfat yogurt	Ice cream
Low-fat or nonfat ricotta cheese	Many sausages
Beans and legumes	Bologna and other cold cuts, unless extra lean
Tofu	

form the structure of body tissues, such as hair, skin, muscles, tendons, and cartilage. *Soluble proteins* form the thousands of different body enzymes (substances that help speed up biochemical reactions in the body), hormones (chemical messengers that control body processes), and proteins in the blood. Blood proteins include hemoglobin, which carries oxygen to cells throughout the body for energy production, and antibodies, which help the body fight disease.

Soluble proteins also maintain several important balances within the body. Proteins in cells help regulate their mineral balance; proteins in the blood help maintain fluid balance. Other soluble proteins help keep a specific pH balance (a measure of acidity or alkalinity) in body systems.

Proteins also help regulate the nervous system. Two amino acids have been found to help transmit nerve impulses. Researchers are investigating how the amino acids in a person's diet may affect behavior and the nervous system.

Finally, proteins can be metabolized to produce energy. The body uses CARBOHYDRATES and fats for energy first, saving proteins for more specialized uses. However, if there are not enough carbohydrates or fats to satisfy energy needs, the body uses protein for this purpose. (See also BODY METABOLISM; ENERGY, FOOD.)

Protein Requirements Most young men need about 45 to 59 grams of protein every day, and young women need about 44 to 46 grams. As people age, they generally need less protein. The average American diet contains about 100 grams of protein daily, or about twice as much as is required. You can roughly calculate your protein needs by dividing your body weight by three. For example, a person who weighs 150 pounds will need about 50 grams of protein per day. To make sure that you get the amount of protein you need, eat two to three servings of foods from the MEAT, POULTRY, DRY BEANS, EGGS, AND NUTS GROUP every day. A serving of meat is 3 ounces (85 grams) cooked; the portion should be about the size of a deck of cards. One-half cup of beans, or one egg, has the protein equivalent of 1 ounce of meat.

RISK FACTORS
▶ ▶ ▶ ▶ ▶ ▶

Even a minor protein deficiency can cause FATIGUE and irritability. It also makes a person more vulnerable to infection because of lowered antibody production. In addition, wounds will heal slowly, and recovery from illness will take longer. Prolonged protein deficiency may result in anemia or liver disorders. Although protein is essential, excessive amounts are not beneficial. Excess proteins are usually converted to fatty acids and stored as BODY FAT.

RISK FACTORS
▶ ▶ ▶ ▶ ▶ ▶

The average American diet generally provides more than enough protein. However, people who follow extreme weight loss diets or who have EATING DISORDERS, such as anorexia nervosa, can have protein deficiencies that eventually lead to MALNUTRITION. Malnutrition caused by protein deficiency is common in developing countries.

· ·

▶ **RECOMMENDED DIETARY ALLOWANCE** The recommended dietary allowance (RDA) is the amount of any essential NUTRIENT that a person should consume daily to maintain good health. The "Percent Daily Value" used in FOOD LABELING, which provides information on the amount of each nutrient contained in one serving of the food, is generally based on the RDA for that nutrient. The RDA is an amount that should meet the needs of most healthy individuals within a particular group.

Because nutritional needs vary by age and sex, so do RDAs. In addition, the special dietary requirements of pregnant and nursing women are taken into consideration. Even within these specific groups, however, the needs of individuals vary. Therefore, the RDA is determined by estimating the average person's need for the nutrient and then increasing that amount to account for the variation in people's nutritional needs. You should also remember that RDAs apply only to healthy people. Disease and environmental stress can increase the body's needs for certain nutrients.

The Food and Nutrition Board of the National Academy of Sciences, which establishes the RDAs, periodically reviews its recommendations for nutrient intake. Currently, RDAs exist for PROTEIN and 18 VITAMINS and MINERALS. However, in 1997, the board began the process of updating RDAs, using a new standard known as *dietary reference intakes* (DRI). The DRIs will combine the RDA with another value, the *adequate intake* or AI. The RDA is a recommended level of a particular nutrient that meets the needs of almost all healthy individuals in the specified age and gender group. The AI, although similar in meaning, is used for nutrients about which there is not enough scientific evidence to create a firm RDA. These revisions have changed the recommendations for some nutrients, but the best way to meet them will remain the same: by eating a variety of healthful foods. (See also DIETARY GUIDELINES.)

▶ REST

Rest is physical and mental relaxation that helps overcome FATIGUE, reduces stress, and restores energy to the body. Adequate rest, including periods of sleep and relaxation, is an important part of a healthy LIFESTYLE.

Relaxation. *Taking a short break from your work or switching to a different activity can help you relax.*

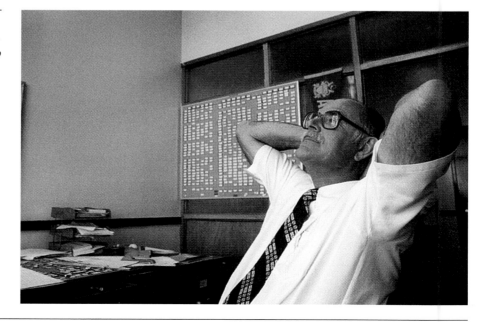

Without enough rest, a person feels tired, lacks concentration, and loses efficiency in physical and mental tasks.

Sleep Sleep allows the body and mind to rest. During sleep, BODY METABOLISM, HEART RATE, and breathing become slower, and body temperature drops. Although requirements differ for each individual, most adults need between 7 and 9 hours of sleep every day.

Relaxation Relaxation involves reducing physical and mental tension, thus lowering *stress*. A sense of physical relaxation often occurs after vigorous exercise, such as jogging or participating in an active sport. There are also several specific techniques for achieving relaxation. These include breathing exercises, progressive muscle relaxation, biofeedback, and meditation.

Breathing exercises consist of slow, deep breaths and emphasize exhaling slowly and gently. These exercises can be performed to aid in relaxation whenever feelings of stress occur. *Progressive muscle relaxation* means alternately tensing and relaxing muscle groups, working progressively (from the feet to the head, for instance) until the whole body is relaxed. A quiet room, a comfortable mat or mattress, and soothing background music can enhance muscle relaxation. *Biofeedback* uses monitoring devices to detect activity and tension within the body. An enhanced awareness of the body can aid relaxation and reduce tension. One biofeedback method, for example, uses small electrodes on the forehead to monitor muscle tension. This equipment provides feedback on whether relaxation techniques have been successful in relaxing muscles. *Meditation* helps a person achieve a relaxed mind and body by combining physical relaxation with concentration on an image or repetitive thought (called a mantra) to block out distracting thoughts and other stimuli.

HEALTHY CHOICES
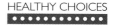

Try to include periods of relaxation in each day. Even a change of pace—something as simple as switching to a different activity for a short time—can help relieve tension.

Recuperation Extra rest is normally beneficial to anyone who is recuperating from illness or injury. A day or two of rest is recommended for most minor sports injuries, for example, followed by a gradual return to activity that gently exercises the injured area. Activity increases blood flow, which speeds healing and helps prevent muscles from weakening and joints from becoming stiff. More serious injuries or illnesses may require longer periods of rest to allow the body to heal. (See also ENERGY, PHYSICAL; SLEEP, 1; RELAXATION TRAINING, 5; SLEEP PROBLEMS, 5; STRESS-MANAGEMENT TECHNIQUES, 5.)

▶ **RISK FACTORS**   Risk factors are characteristics or behaviors that increase the likelihood of medical disorders or diseases. Some risk factors, such as those having to do with age, sex, race, and hereditary characteristics, are beyond an individual's control. However, others, such as a dangerous environment or an inactive lifestyle, are largely controllable.

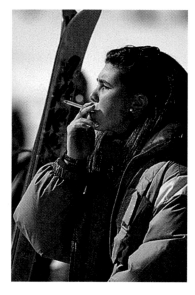

Risk Factors. *Cigarette smoking is a behavioral risk factor that contributes directly to lung cancer, heart disease, and other illnesses.*

Risk Factors That Cannot Be Controlled   The traits and qualities that people inherit from their parents are beyond their control. One of those traits is the tendency to develop certain diseases. For example, a person whose mother and father had heart disease or cancer has a greater chance of developing that disease than a person who has no such family history. No one can do anything to reduce inherited risk factors. However, if people are aware of these inherited tendencies, they can work harder to control other risk factor areas, such as environment and lifestyle.

Risk Factors That Can Be Controlled   A person's environment is controllable to some extent. For example, although people cannot change the air they breathe, they may be able to move out of a neighborhood or region where the air quality is poor.

LIFESTYLE, a critical factor in a person's health, is also one of the easiest to control. The way people live can greatly increase or decrease their risk of developing diseases. Behaviors such as smoking cigarettes, eating a diet high in saturated FATS and CHOLESTEROL, and failing to EXERCISE regularly can all contribute to heart disease. The greater the number of these risk factors, the greater the likelihood of contracting the disease.

Several diseases, including heart disease and many forms of cancer, have risk factors that are based on behaviors and habits related to diet and exercise. Appropriate changes in environment and lifestyle can reduce or entirely eliminate many risk factors.

Controlling Risk Factors   An awareness of the risk factors for various diseases is the first step toward making behavioral changes that can reduce the likelihood of becoming ill. For example, by knowing that cigarette smoking, a high-fat diet, and excessive alcohol consumption are major risk factors in cancer, a person can choose to stop smoking, eat a low-fat diet, and keep alcohol use to a minimum in order to lessen the risk of developing it. Some lifestyle changes, such as eating a diet rich in fruits, vegetables, and whole grains, can reduce the risk of many diseases.

People who already have a disease can also take action to control risk factors that could make it worse. People who have diabetes can control their diet and weight and avoid smoking. If they do not control these risk factors, their disease will probably get much worse. (See also FITNESS; MALNUTRITION; OVERWEIGHT; HEREDITY AND ENVIRONMENT, **5**.)

▶ RUNNING

Running is a popular exercise activity because it is a convenient way to burn calories and increase fitness. The only special equipment it requires is a good pair of running shoes. A form of AEROBIC EXERCISE, running improves the fitness of the heart and lungs and strengthens the muscles of the lower body. Participation in running varies from casually jogging short distances around the neighborhood to competing in 26.2-mile (about 42.2-km) *marathon* races.

HEALTHY CHOICES

Benefits of Running   Like all aerobic exercises, running improves *cardiovascular fitness*. The positive effects of a regular running program include lower blood pressure and a slower heart rate. Running is also one of the most effective exercises for burning calories and reducing weight. A

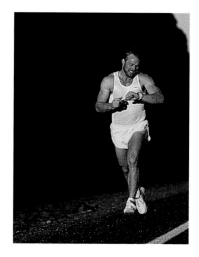

Clothing for Running. *If you plan to run where there is traffic, wear bright-colored clothing. If you run at night, wear clothing with reflective strips that can be seen easily.*

runner can expend 400 or more calories in half an hour. These effects can be achieved by a half-hour run taken 3 or 4 days each week. Regular running improves BODY COMPOSITION by adding some muscle mass while substantially decreasing BODY FAT.

Preparing to Run If you are new to running, begin by taking brisk walks for 30 to 45 minutes, three times a week. Move on to alternately walking and running, gradually increasing the amount of time spent running. Begin each running session with 5 to 10 minutes of warm-up and STRETCHING EXERCISES to loosen muscles. End each session with a cool-down period of brisk walking to allow your blood pressure and heart rate to return to normal.

A runner's most important purchase is a pair of high-quality running shoes. Running shoes should feel comfortable and give good support. Especially important are a well-cushioned heel, a flexible midsole, and plenty of room above the toe. If your foot is between sizes, buy the size that is slightly too big. If your foot rolls excessively inward (pronation) or outward (supination), pain and injuries can result. Special devices (called orthotics) prescribed by foot doctors can help correct foot roll. (See also ATHLETIC FOOTWEAR.)

Running Safety Runners put a great deal of stress on their legs, knees, and feet. Most injuries can be prevented by wearing the proper shoes, avoiding hard or uneven running surfaces, and increasing running time gradually. The most common injuries are blisters, ankle sprains, shin-splints (pain in the shins), and muscle pulls and cramps.

Pay attention to your body's signals, and give injuries time to heal. Any pain or tenderness that does not clear up, or that recurs, should be investigated by a specialist in SPORTS MEDICINE or an orthopedist (bone doctor). (See also ENDURANCE; FITNESS; HEART RATE; SPORTS INJURIES.)

▶ SALT

Unsalty Snacks. *Many traditionally salty foods are now available in low-salt or salt-free varieties.*

Salt, or sodium chloride, is a mineral that is widely used to season and preserve foods. It is a compound of two MINERALS, SODIUM and *chloride*. Essential to good health, these minerals help to balance the level of water

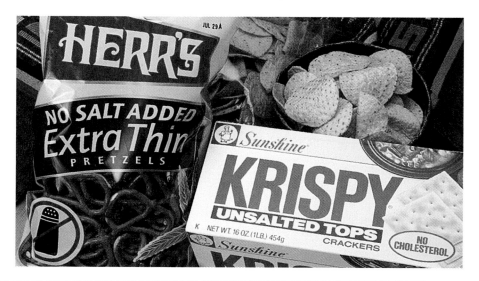

in the body. Like POTASSIUM, sodium is an *electrolyte*. Electrolytes transmit electrical currents that enable nerve impulses to travel between cells.

Most table salt is iodized, meaning that small amounts of *iodine* have been added to it. Iodine is necessary to regulate the activity of the thyroid gland. The use of iodized salt prevents iodine deficiency, which can cause an enlargement of the thyroid gland called *goiter.*

RISK FACTORS
▶ ▶ ▶ ▶ ▶ ▶

HEALTHY CHOICES
◆●●●●●●●●●●●●

Most Americans consume more salt than they need. For sodium-sensitive people, too much of this mineral increases the risk of *hypertension,* or high blood pressure. Sodium sensitivity seems to run in families. In order to reduce sodium intake, many people substitute seasonings that do not contain sodium. (See also FOOD ADDITIVES; POTASSIUM; HYPERTENSION, **3**.)

SNACKING

A snack is any food that is eaten between meals. Some people do not choose to eat snacks at all, while others make them a major part of their diet, eating several small meals each day instead of three large ones. Teenagers, who have high energy needs, are especially likely to snack to maintain their energy throughout the day. The more snacks you consume, the more important it is to choose nutritious snack foods.

Types of Snacks   When people think of snack foods, they often think of so-called "junk food," or ready-to-eat packaged foods that are typically high in CALORIES, FATS, SALT, or SUGAR and low in other NUTRIENTS. Such foods include potato chips, candy, cookies, and soft drinks. While these foods can be part of a healthy diet when eaten in moderation, filling up on them may prevent you from eating other, more nutritious foods.

HEALTHY CHOICES
◆●●●●●●●●●●●●

Healthful snacks supply nutrients as well as energy. Quick, healthful snacks include fresh fruits, raw vegetables, nuts, seeds, cereal, yogurt, cheese slices, and unbuttered popcorn. Although some of these are high in fats, they provide more VITAMINS, MINERALS, and PROTEIN than do most typical snack foods. Fruits, vegetables, and grains also contain FIBER, which fills you up and satisfies your APPETITE until your next meal.

HEALTHY CHOICES
◆●●●●●●●●●●●●

Guidelines for Snacking   To make snacks part of a balanced diet, try to choose nutritious snacks most of the time. This may mean planning ahead to have fresh fruit or a sandwich available, rather than relying on packaged foods from vending machines. When only prepackaged foods are available, choose baked snacks (such as unsalted pretzels) instead of fried snacks (such as most potato chips). Look for foods that are made from whole-grain flour instead of white flour.

Recently, many manufacturers of packaged snack foods have begun to reduce the fat content of some of their snacks. Products such as fat-free cookies and potato chips that are baked, rather than fried, have become extremely popular. However, such foods may supply as many calories as the original versions, or even more, and they may be higher in sugar and salt. Always read the nutrition label on packaged products to determine how many calories they contain and how many of those calories come from fat. (See also DIET FOOD; FOOD LABELING.)

Although the quality of the food you eat is most important, be aware of the quantity as well. If you eat snack foods directly from a large package, it is easy to consume large amounts without realizing it. Also, eating many snacks without reducing the size of your meals will almost certainly cause a weight gain. Therefore, it is important to remember to include snacks when calculating your food consumption for the day. (See also FAST FOOD; FOOD GUIDE PYRAMID; WEIGHT MANAGEMENT.)

▶ SODIUM

Sodium is an essential MINERAL that performs a number of important functions in the body. Along with POTASSIUM and other substances, it helps transport electric charges between nerves and muscles and maintains a balance of fluids in the body. Sodium is also involved in the proper functioning of muscles, including the heart. Although sodium is most familiar as a component of table SALT, it is found in almost all natural and processed foods.

The main forms of sodium found in food are sodium chloride (table salt), sodium bicarbonate (baking soda), and monosodium glutamate (MSG), a flavor enhancer used in some prepared or packaged foods. Large amounts of sodium are present in many cheeses, breads and cereals, cured and smoked meats, pickles, bacon, and snack foods. Processed and packaged foods tend to be especially high in sodium, even when they do not taste particularly salty. Ketchup is just one example. Sodium also occurs naturally in vegetables such as spinach, celery, beets, carrots, and cabbage. Some drugs, including many *laxatives* and *sedatives,* also contain sodium, as does drinking water that has been treated with softeners.

Because sodium occurs in almost all foods, most Americans consume much more of it than they need (see illustration: High Sodium Content in Processed Foods). In fact, the average American consumes two to three times the recommended amount each day. Too much sodium in the diet causes the body to retain water, and in some people, this can result in swelling of the legs and dizziness. It may also increase the risk of

RISK FACTORS
▶ ▶ ▶ ▶ ▶ ▶

High Sodium Content in Processed Foods. *Foods that are high in sodium do not always taste salty, so a salt-sensitive consumer should check food labels.*

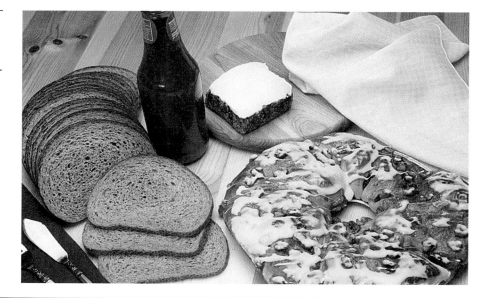

hypertension, or high blood pressure, although recent studies indicate that this risk is significant only for certain sodium-sensitive individuals. In addition, too much sodium in the diet may weaken bones because sodium removes CALCIUM from the body when it is excreted.

Sodium deficiency, however, can also be dangerous. Persistent diarrhea or vomiting, excessive sweating, kidney disease, disorders of the adrenal glands, and prolonged treatment with *diuretic drugs* (which increase the output of urine) can all result in sodium loss. (See also DEHYDRATION; DIURETIC, **7.**)

HEALTHY CHOICES

No official RECOMMENDED DIETARY ALLOWANCE has been established for sodium. However, the American Heart Association advises that adults consume no more than 2400 milligrams per day, or the amount in about 1¼ teaspoon (6 ml) of salt. This amount includes both the salt already present in foods and table salt that is added to foods at home. People with high blood pressure, kidney or liver disease, or edema (an abnormal fluid buildup in the body) as well as those who are at risk for these conditions should follow a *low-sodium diet.* Most fresh, unprocessed foods are naturally low in salt. People who want to cut down on sodium should check the sodium content listed on the nutrition labels of packaged foods and take the salt shaker off the table; herbs and spices can provide just as much flavor as table salt. (See also FOOD ADDITIVES; VITAMINS; WATER; HYPERTENSION, **3.**)

▶ SPORTS AND FITNESS

Sports and fitness are interrelated. Fitness improves performance levels in most sports; regular participation in many sports improves fitness by one or more of several basic measures. The primary measures of FITNESS include STRENGTH, muscular and cardiovascular ENDURANCE, and FLEXIBILITY. The nature and degree of fitness benefits vary with each sport and the level at which a sport is played.

Choosing a Sport   For the competitive athlete, excellence and victory are the goals of sports. For most people, however, improving fitness, having fun with friends, and the thrill of competing and winning are the goals of sports. People who exercise to achieve fitness should choose a sport they enjoy that also matches their fitness goals. For example, for *cardiovascular endurance* and strength, CYCLING, SWIMMING, and roller-skating are good choices. If strength and flexibility are your goals, gymnastics and karate are among the better choices.

The choice of a sport may also depend on many other factors, including your body type, fitness level, and personality as well as the climate where you live. In addition, you will want to find a sport that fits your schedule and that you can afford.

If your sport of choice is seasonal, you may want to take up a second one in order to stay fit all year. For example, you might ski cross-country in the winter and play tennis during the rest of the year. A mix of enjoyable activities provides variety and helps you stay challenged and interested. In addition, if you choose sports that emphasize different elements of fitness, your program will be more balanced. You will

Sport	Aerobic fitness	Upper-body strength	Lower-body strength	Muscle endurance	Flexibility
Baseball	1	2	2	1	3
Basketball	4	2	2	2	4
Football, touch	2	2	2	2	3
Golf	2	1	1	1	2
Hockey	4	3	3	2	3
Martial arts	4	4	3	3	4
Skiing, downhill	3	2	3	4	3
Soccer	4	2	2	2	3
Tennis	3	1	2	1	3
Volleyball	2	2	2	2	3

SPORTS AND FITNESS REQUIREMENTS

Scale: 1=low; 2=moderate; 3=above average; 4=high

also place less stress on any single part of your body, minimizing your chance of injury.

Individual Sports Some people prefer individual sports, those in which they can participate alone or with one or two others. They may enjoy the solitude of rowing after a hectic day or the challenge of trying to better their last golf score.

Individual sports come in many varieties and offer a wide range of fitness benefits. For example, AEROBIC DANCE, martial arts, RUNNING, cross-country skiing, and brisk WALKING all build cardiovascular fitness. In addition, martial arts build strength and flexibility; the others build *muscular endurance*. Strength is the major fitness benefit of downhill skiing and weight lifting.

Team Sports Some people prefer team sports. They may enjoy the strategy, competition, and teamwork involved or the camaraderie associated with practices and games.

The fitness benefits of team sports vary. For example, basketball, ice hockey, field hockey, lacrosse, racquetball, and soccer build cardiovascular and muscular endurance as well as flexibility. Football builds strength; baseball and softball build strength and flexibility. Many team sports mix rapid bursts of intense exertion with periods of lower intensity.

Getting Started Whether you choose an individual activity or a team sport, you will need to plan and organize your fitness activities. How you begin depends on your level of fitness, how skilled you already are at the sport, the demands the sport makes on your body, and the need for equipment, partners, team members, or a coach. For example, touch football does not require much skill or equipment, but you have to have enough people to make up teams. Fencing, on the other hand, demands a high level of cardiovascular fitness and skill as well as special equipment and a partner.

Training for Sports Before you can train for a sport, you need to analyze its fitness requirements (see chart: Sports and Fitness Requirements). For example, football and baseball require a high degree of upper-body strength, so training for those sports places emphasis on building that area. Sports such as basketball and hockey that demand a great deal of cardiovascular endurance would call for AEROBIC EXERCISE training to improve the body's ability to sustain activity.

After you have analyzed a sport's fitness requirements, you can begin practicing and training. Practicing improves skills that are specific to your sport, such as dribbling in basketball. Training improves your general fitness level so you are better able to excel at any sport. One of the keys to effective training is three good aerobic workouts a week. You should also add strength exercises and STRETCHING EXERCISES. These build overall strength and flexibility and reduce your chances of a sports-related injury.

When you practice or train, be sure to include warm-up and stretching sessions so that your muscles are warm and loose. Afterward, cool down to avoid soreness and aches. As a general rule, make stretching exercises part of every warm-up and cooldown. (See also FITNESS TRAINING; SPORTS INJURIES.)

▶ **SPORTS INJURIES** Every athletic activity carries some risk of injury. This risk varies from sport to sport and with the level of competition. The more physical strain a sport places on the body, the more likely a sports injury is to result. In addition, the nature of individual sports makes certain kinds of injuries more likely than others. Runners, for example, tend to damage their feet, ankles, and legs, whereas tennis players frequently hurt their elbows. The treatment of sports injuries depends on their nature and severity.

Treating Common Sports Injuries Many mild sports injuries, including muscle strains and pulls, bruises, and sprains, can be treated at home with a simple first-aid routine called RICE. RICE stands for **R**est, **I**ce (put ice on the injured area to prevent swelling), **C**ompression (compress the injured area with a bandage), and **E**levation (raise the injured area above the level of the heart to help fluids drain). Treat moderate injuries with the RICE routine for 48 hours. If the injury does not improve in that time, consult a physician. Do not attempt to treat severe sports injuries and serious heat injuries, such as heat exhaustion and heatstroke. Instead, contact a physician immediately. (See also EXERCISE AND HEAT INJURY.)

CONSULT A PHYSICIAN

The following list includes some of the most common sports injuries and how to treat them. (see illustration: Common Sports Injuries)

> ▶ *Back pain and injuries* are a risk in many types of sports. Medical treatments may include medications to relieve pain and relax

muscles; heat treatments; and use of a neck brace. (See also BACK PROBLEMS, **3**.)

▸ *Blisters* form as a result of friction against the skin. They often occur on the foot. A blister should be covered with a thick bandage or a blister pad. Treat broken blisters with an antiseptic. Never break a blister on purpose. (See also BLISTER, **3**.)

▸ *Bruises* result from an impact that causes bleeding under the skin. Treat them with the RICE routine. If pain persists for 3 days, see a physician.

CONSULT A
PHYSICIAN

▸ *Chafing* is rawness and irritation of the skin. It frequently occurs in the groin area. Treat chafing with a medicated powder, and prevent further problems by wearing cotton clothing.

RISK FACTORS
▸ ▸ ▸ ▸ ▸ ▸

▸ *Cramps* are caused by muscle spasms and are more likely when the athlete has not warmed up completely before exercising. If a cramp occurs, stop exercising right away, stretch the muscle, and drink plenty of fluids.

▸ *Foot injuries,* such as heel bruises, are usually caused by sudden and severe impact of the foot on a hard surface. To treat them, use the RICE routine. For heel bruises, wear a heel pad when putting weight on the heel again. (See also FOOT PROBLEMS, **3**.)

▸ *Head injuries* should always be treated by a doctor. A blow to the head can result in a *concussion,* an injury to the brain when it is shaken inside the skull. A player who returns to a sport too soon after receiving a concussion is extremely vulnerable to further injury. Repeated concussions can cause permanent brain damage. (See also CONCUSSION, **8**.)

▸ *Knee injuries,* such as "runner's knee" (a dull, aching pain caused by overuse) require rest and, in many cases, specialized medical care.

▸ *Lacerations* and *abrasions,* more commonly referred to as cuts and scrapes, can often be treated with simple first aid. Wash the affected area with an antiseptic, and cover it with a bandage or dressing. A tetanus shot may be necessary if dirt or other foreign matter has entered the wound. If the injury is severe, or if an infection develops, see a physician. (See also INFECTION, **2**; TETANUS, **2**.)

CONSULT A
PHYSICIAN

▸ *Shinsplints* are an aching pain on the front of the lower legs. This is a common problem that is often caused by incorrect movements, poor shoes, or a very hard exercise surface. Shinsplints usually improve with rest.

▸ *Sore muscles* often occur 8 to 10 hours after strenuous exercise. To treat them, keep muscles moving with slow, easy stretches. You can relieve the pain with over-the-counter painkillers, such as aspirin or acetaminophen; warm baths; and massage. Children or teenagers should not, however, be given aspirin. (See also ANALGESICS, **7**.)

▸ *Sprains* and *strains* can be mild to severe. Mild sprains and strains cause tenderness but no swelling and can be treated with RICE. Moderate sprains and strains limit function and cause tenderness, pain, swelling, discoloration, and possible muscle spasms. Use the RICE routine at first. If the affected area has not improved after 24 to 72 hours, see a physician. For severe sprains and strains, call a physician immediately. (See also SPRAINS AND STRAINS, **8**.)

CONSULT A
PHYSICIAN

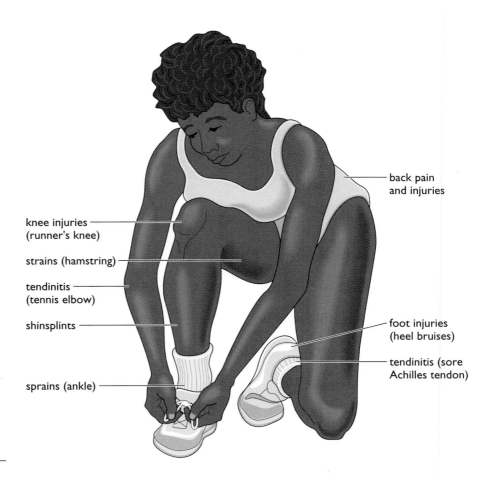

back pain
and injuries

knee injuries
(runner's knee)

strains (hamstring)

tendinitis
(tennis elbow)

shinsplints

foot injuries
(heel bruises)

tendinitis (sore
Achilles tendon)

sprains (ankle)

Common Sports Injuries.

CONSULT A
PHYSICIAN

▶ *Tendinitis,* or an inflamed tendon, often occurs in the Achilles tendon behind the ankle, the shoulder joint, and the elbow (resulting in tennis elbow). Treatment includes the RICE routine and resting for a few weeks, or until the pain subsides. See a physician if you think that you might have torn a tendon or if you have had repeated problems with tendinitis. (See also TENDINITIS, **3.**)

Tips for Preventing Sports Injuries Many injuries that occur as a result of exercise can be prevented. A large proportion of sports injuries are the result of exercising too little or too often or increasing your training level too fast. Weekend athletes who have no regular FITNESS routine, for example, frequently overextend themselves when they do take part in a sport, and they get hurt as a result. At the other extreme, competitive athletes need to be careful not to risk injury as the result of overtraining. Moderation is a key to avoiding sports injuries.

Be realistic about how much you can do when you begin a sport or exercise regimen. First, assess your physical ability and condition; then choose activities that suit your body. For example, if you have knee problems, you should not take up CYCLING or soccer.

HEALTHY CHOICES

Learn as much as you can about the injury risks of the sports you take part in. Some sports that are popular with young people, such as football, soccer, and basketball, can be hard on joints and may lead to problems and injuries later in life. Be sure to use all necessary safety equipment. Many sports require, for instance, that people wear good shock-absorbing shoes to prevent pain and injuries. Always buy the highest-quality equipment that you can afford. In addition, select appropriate places to exercise. For example, a resilient surface is important for cushioning the impact of running, jumping, or doing aerobics.

Condition your body thoroughly by planning a balanced EXERCISE program. In addition, focus on building strong muscles around the joints that receive the most strain in your sport. If you experience pain at any time during your workout, stop immediately and rest.

Warm up and stretch muscles thoroughly for at least 10 minutes before exercising. This increases the temperature of your muscles so that they are more flexible and harder to injure. After exercising, cool down gradually to let your HEART RATE and muscles return to a resting state.

RISK FACTORS
▶ ▶ ▶ ▶ ▶ ▶

If possible, avoid extremes in temperature. Strenuous exercise during hot, humid weather can lead to heatstroke or other heat-related problems. In cold weather, muscles can be strained more easily. (See also ATHLETIC FOOTWEAR; SPORTS MEDICINE; STRENGTH TRAINING; STRETCHING EXERCISE; PAIN, 3; FIRST AID, 8; INJURIES; 8; RICE, 8.)

- -

▶ **SPORTS MEDICINE**   Sports medicine is a rapidly growing medical field that specializes in improving FITNESS, treating and preventing SPORTS INJURIES, and providing physical rehabilitation for injured athletes. Treatment of an injury may include an exercise program, nutritional advice, fitness tests, or surgical repair of damaged tissues.

Sports Medicine Specialists   The first sports medicine specialists were team physicians who provided medical care for amateur and professional sports teams. Today, many sports medicine specialists operate *sports medicine clinics* where both team athletes and those who engage in individual sports, such as RUNNING or CYCLING, can seek treatment for injuries.

The need for sports medicine specialists stems from the fact that the physical demands of specific sports tend to cause specific kinds of injuries. The torn rotator cuff muscles in the shoulders of baseball pitchers and the torn knee ligaments of running backs in football are two common examples. Some injuries are so closely associated with a sport that they take their name from it; for example, runner's knee and tennis elbow are recognized medical conditions. Many of these injuries and conditions are rare in nonathletes and may be unfamiliar to the nonspecialist.

Many doctors who practice sports medicine are *orthopedists* or orthopedic surgeons, specialists in treating disorders of the musculoskeletal system. Some *podiatrists* (foot specialists) also treat athletes. Both they and orthopedists may provide advice on ATHLETIC FOOTWEAR and prescribe *orthotic devices*. These are foam, leather, or plastic inserts worn in the shoe to correct foot abnormalities. A few *osteopathic physicians* (D.O.'s) specialize in sports medicine.

Some sports medicine practitioners are not physicians. *Chiropractors* treat injuries by manipulating the muscles, joints, and spine. Physical therapists and athletic trainers plan exercise and treatment programs for injured athletes. A relatively new type of sports medicine practitioners,

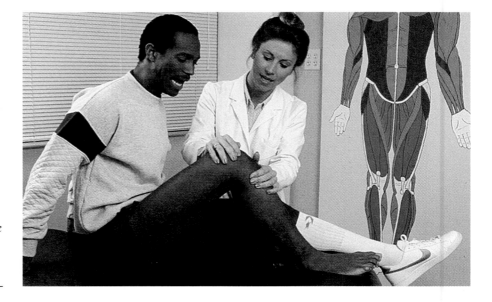

Treating Sports Injuries. *In a sports medicine clinic, one or more specialists may advise an athlete about healing an existing injury or preventing future problems.*

sports psychologists, deal with the mental and emotional aspects of athletic performance. Many sports injuries can also be helped by massage therapy and alternative therapies such as *acupuncture,* used to relieve pain.

Treating and Preventing Sports Injuries Most competitive athletes want to continue to participate in their sports while their injuries are healing. When an athlete must take a break from a sport, treatment may include alternative forms of activity so that the athlete can keep fit while resting the injured body part. An injured runner, for example, might row, swim, or lift weights while a leg injury heals.

An important emphasis in sports medicine is the building of STRENGTH, ENDURANCE, and FLEXIBILITY as a means of preventing sports injuries. Clinic physicians also provide advice about clothing, equipment, and technique to help athletes avoid injuries. (See also ACUPUNCTURE, **3**; ALTERNATIVE HEALTH CARE, **9**; CHIROPRACTOR, **9**; OSTEOPATHIC PHYSICIANS (D.O.'S), **9**; PHYSICAL THERAPIST, **9**; PHYSICIANS (M.D.'S): Orthopedist, **9**; PODIATRIST, **9**.)

▶ SPORTS NUTRITION

Sports nutrition refers to the particular nutritional needs of people who participate regularly in athletics. While both athletes and nonathletes require the same basic NUTRIENTS (CARBOHYDRATES, PROTEINS, FATS, VITAMINS, MINERALS, and WATER) athletes may need more of certain nutrients in order to sustain their best efforts.

HEALTHY CHOICES
••••••••••••

Energy Needs Because carbohydrates are the body's main energy source, athletes will find it helpful to eat foods rich in complex carbohydrates, such as breads, pasta, potatoes, rice, and cereals. The digestive process breaks down these carbohydrates and changes them to GLUCOSE, which circulates in the bloodstream. The body's cells use some of this glucose immediately to produce energy. The body stores the rest in the form of *glycogen* in muscles and in the liver or in the form of BODY FAT.

When athletes need energy, their bodies use both glycogen and fat. High-intensity activities, such as sprinting, draw mainly on glycogen for energy. Activities requiring ENDURANCE, such as long-distance running, draw on both glycogen and stored fat. The amount of energy an athlete needs depends not only on the activity but also on the individual athlete's body weight and physical condition.

Athletes do have slightly higher protein needs than nonathletes. However, since most Americans get more protein than they need in their normal diet, consuming extra protein is generally not necessary. A BALANCED DIET should also provide enough vitamins and minerals.

Fluid Needs An adequate amount of water in the body is essential both to top physical performance and to general good health. Water, as a major component of blood, transports oxygen, glucose, and other nutrients to body cells. It also helps to remove waste products.

RISK FACTORS
▶ ▶ ▶ ▶ ▶ ▶

Strenuous or prolonged physical activity can cause the body to lose large amounts of water through perspiration. As the body's fluid level drops, physical performance declines. When the body's water level gets too low, DEHYDRATION is said to occur, and an athlete may experience such symptoms as fatigue, muscle cramps, and extreme thirst. (See also EXERCISE AND HEAT INJURY.)

Timing Proper sports nutrition means not only *what* athletes eat and drink, but *when*. For example, to prevent dehydration, athletes cannot wait until they feel thirsty to drink liquids. Athletes should drink at least 2 cups (0.47 L) of water, juice, milk, or a sports drink a couple of hours before their sports activity. Just before participating, they should drink 2 more cups; they should then make it a point to drink ½ cup (0.12 L) every 15 minutes during and after the activity. Additional liquid may be needed in very hot weather.

HEALTHY CHOICES
▪▪▪▪▪▪▪▪▪▪▪▪▪

Planning ahead applies to food intake, too. For example, trained athletes who intend to take part in a sports event that requires endurance often increase their intake of carbohydrates several days before the event. Such *carbohydrate loading* enables the body to store extra glycogen, which will then be available as an energy source. Carbohydrate loading is not recommended for children or teenagers, however.

▶ **STARCH**

Starch is a complex CARBOHYDRATE, the body's primary source of energy from food. Starches consist of a long chemical chain of simple SUGARS linked together. Foods high in starch, such as grains and certain vegetables, often contain large amounts of FIBER as well. Both starches and fiber are called *polysaccharides,* meaning "many sugars," for their chemical structure.

Nutritional Value of Starch Complex carbohydrates are excellent foods for two reasons. First, they produce energy for the body in a form that is broken down more slowly than simple carbohydrates (sugars). More important, starchy foods, which are entirely of plant origin, are usually rich in VITAMINS, MINERALS, PROTEINS, and fiber and low in FAT. For these reasons,

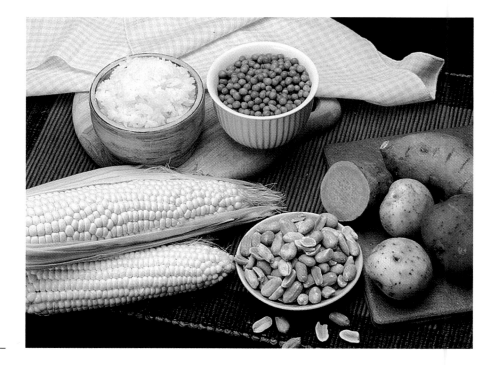

Foods High in Starch. *Nutrition experts recommend that the largest percentage of total daily calories come from complex carbohydrates, found in foods from plant sources such as those shown here.*

nutritionists recommend that 55 to 60 percent of a person's caloric intake be in the form of carbohydrates, mostly complex carbohydrates.

During the digestive process, starches are broken down into simple sugars called *monosaccharides* ("one sugar unit"). These are absorbed by the body and converted into GLUCOSE, the fuel of cell metabolism. If there is excess glucose, a small amount is stored in the liver and muscles as glycogen for later use. The remainder is converted into BODY FAT.

Sources of Starch   The best source of starch is grains, such as rice, wheat, and corn. The legume family (beans and peas) and the tuber family (potatoes, yams, and cassava) are also good sources of starch (see illustration: Foods High in Starch). (See also BREAD, CEREAL, RICE, AND PASTA GROUP; VEGETABLE GROUP; ENERGY, FOOD.)

HEALTHY CHOICES

▶ **STRENGTH**

Strength is the amount of force muscles can exert against resistance. Adequate strength helps the body meet the physical demands of everyday life. It can prevent injuries, help avoid muscle aches and pains, and improve posture, among other benefits. Strength, FLEXIBILITY, and muscular and cardiovascular ENDURANCE are the basic elements of physical FITNESS.

Strength can be increased with regular EXERCISE that places demands on muscles. When muscles work hard against resistance, they break down slightly and then rebuild themselves, becoming larger and stronger. Without regular exercise, however, strength decreases, and muscles *atrophy* (grow smaller), especially as an adult grows older.

Measuring Strength   Specific exercises are a simple way to measure overall strength. The amount of weight a person can lift is the best

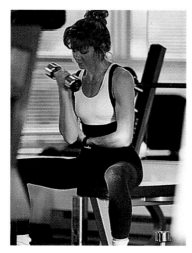

Building Strength. *Strength is an important part of fitness. Developing upper-body strength, for example, can greatly improve the performance of long-distance runners.*

indication of strength. However, attempting to lift as much weight as possible can be dangerous, especially for beginners. Therefore, strength is usually judged by an exercise that requires moving a lighter weight as many times as possible, such as push-ups. Although this test actually measures muscular endurance, it is also a reasonable indication of the strength of chest and arm muscles.

Increasing Strength A program of STRENGTH TRAINING builds up muscles by placing progressively greater resistance against them. Working with weights, whether using EXERCISE MACHINES or free weights, is a common and effective method of improving strength.

Strength training requires regular workouts: usually three times a week with at least a day of rest between workouts to prevent muscle fatigue, soreness, and injury. Generally, strength exercises are performed in "sets." A set is several consecutive repetitions (usually 8 to 12 without resting) of an exercise that places a great deal of resistance against a specific muscle group. With regular repetition, muscles should respond to this kind of training by becoming stronger. As the exercise becomes easier with increasing strength, you can also increase the amount of resistance used in the exercise, either by adding more weight or by doing more sets. This keeps the muscles working hard, the key to building strength. (See also MUSCLE, **1**.)

▶ **STRENGTH TRAINING** Strength training is exercise that builds up the muscles and increases the body's ability to perform work. All strength exercises force a muscle or muscle group to contract against resistance—for example, by lifting a weight. Strength training is based on three principles: *overload,* or pushing the muscles beyond their normal limits; *progression,* or adding weight or repetitions as strength and endurance improve; and *balance,* or developing all muscle groups equally.

Strength training improves both STRENGTH and muscular ENDURANCE. In addition to building muscle mass, it strengthens connective tissue, such as the tendons and ligaments that join muscles and bones together. Strength training with weights can also increase bone mass, which may help prevent *osteoporosis,* the loss of bone mass that often occurs in older people. The three basic kinds of strength training are isometric exercise, isotonic exercise, and isokinetic exercise.

HEALTHY CHOICES
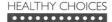

Isometric Exercise In isometric exercise, a person pushes against an immovable object, such as a wall or doorway, or pushes muscle groups against each other. Each muscle contraction is held for 5 to 8 seconds, and then the muscle is relaxed. Isometric exercise is not favored as a means of developing overall strength because it exercises a muscle in only one position; also, it raises blood pressure in some individuals. Isometric exercise can be useful, however, for people who want to build strength at a specific point in the range of motion; for example, it is often used in rehabilitation after a joint injury. In this type of exercise, the joint does not move and is therefore not stressed.

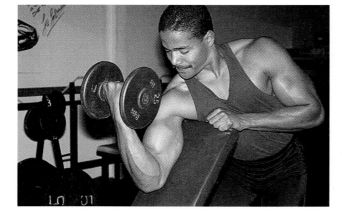

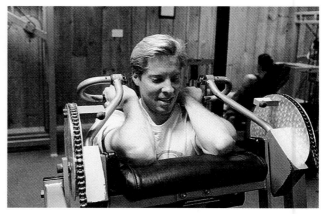

Types of Strength Training.
Weight lifting is a type of isotonic exercise in which the arm muscles lift weights as they move through a range of motion. Isokinetic exercise works in a similar way but uses special machines.

Isotonic Exercise   Isotonic exercise works by making a muscle push a weight through a range of motion. To increase strength most efficiently, the weight should be near the maximum a person can push or lift, and the number of repetitions should be low. Doing more repetitions of a given exercise using less weight, by contrast, will build endurance.

While weight lifting is the best-known type of isotonic exercise, devices such as flexible rubber tubes and bands can also be used for this type of exercise. Instead of a weight, the stretching of the rubber provides resistance for the muscle to work against. Many calisthenic exercises, such as push-ups and chin-ups, are also isotonic.

Isokinetic Exercise   Isokinetic exercise also requires muscles to lift a weight through a range of motion. It is performed on EXERCISE MACHINES (such as Nautilus and Cybex) that use cables, pulleys, weights, and other devices to control the speed of the motion throughout the exercise. In this way the machine keeps a maximum load on the muscle throughout its movement.

Using Strength Exercise   At the beginning of a strength training program, it is wise to work with a trainer or physical education teacher to establish an exercise routine, set up a workout schedule, and learn proper technique. Each session should start with 5 to 10 minutes of warm-up exercise. After your workout, allow for a brief cooldown period as well. Finally, be sure to rest each group of muscles at least a full day between workout sessions.

Some kinds of strength exercise, especially calisthenics, weight lifting, and isometrics, can be performed at home, using either no special equipment or fairly inexpensive equipment, such as *free weights* (dumbbells or barbells) or rubber exercise tubes and bands. Heavy weight lifting, however, should not be done alone. Do this type of exercise with a partner, or spotter, who can step in and help if you lose control of the weights.

Weight training on machines involves exercising a different muscle group at each machine station. Some weight trainers circuit-train, which means that they move quickly from one station to the next. By greatly reducing the resting time between exercises, *circuit training* raises a person's HEART RATE, providing some aerobic conditioning. Because most strength-building machines are expensive, joining a health club, recreation center, or gym may be necessary. Remember, however, that strength training does little to improve the function of the heart and lungs. It should be combined with AEROBIC EXERCISE and STRETCHING EXERCISE to attain maximum FITNESS. (See also BODYBUILDING; FITNESS TRAINING.)

▶ STRETCHING EXERCISE

Stretching exercise is movement designed to relieve muscle tension and increase FLEXIBILITY. It increases the blood supply to the muscles and other tissues, making them more supple and efficient, which helps prevent injuries such as tears and sprains. Stretching exercise should always be a part of the WARM-UP AND COOLDOWN activities performed before and after other kinds of exercises. By relaxing tight, bunched muscles, stretching is also a good way to improve posture, relieve muscle pain, and even manage stress.

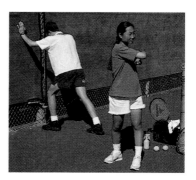

Stretching Leg Muscles. *You can use static stretching to stretch your leg muscles, either by lying on a flat surface or standing against a wall for support.*

Types of Stretching Exercise There are three basic types of stretching techniques.

- *Static stretching* involves stretching a muscle slowly and gently to its limit, holding it there for a time, and then relaxing it.
- *Contract-relax stretching* is a variation of static stretching in which pairs of muscles are alternately stretched and relaxed. First, one muscle is contracted against resistance, such as an object or an exercise partner. As that muscle relaxes, the opposing muscle is contracted. Contract-relax stretching is the best way to improve muscle flexibility.
- In *ballistic stretching,* a person stretches a muscle to its limit and then makes repetitive bouncing movements. This type of stretch is not recommended. It is ineffective and can cause muscle tears and soreness.

Doing Stretching Exercises Stretching exercise, even when part of a warm-up routine, should be preceded by a few minutes of activity to increase blood flow and raise muscle temperature. Walking or jogging in place for a few minutes is a good warm-up before stretching. Stretching during the cooldown period helps develop flexibility efficiently because the muscles are warm and can be stretched more.

Begin each exercise by stretching slowly and smoothly until you feel a mild pull. Then hold the stretch for 15 to 30 seconds. (You can begin with a shorter amount of time and increase duration as you progress.) Breathe slowly and deeply, stretching farther while exhaling. Release the muscle, then repeat the stretch several times. You can improve flexibility by performing a routine of stretching exercises three to five times per week. A good stretching session should last 10 to 30 minutes.

Developing a Stretching Program There are hundreds of different kinds of stretches that can be performed to exercise individual muscles and muscle groups. Exercise and fitness books and magazines can provide instructions on a variety of exercises. You can develop your own stretching program by selecting sets of exercises that are designed to stretch the muscles you want to use. A runner, for example, would perform exercises that stretch the thighs, calves, Achilles tendon, and torso muscles.

Done improperly, however, stretching exercise can cause injuries. For example, locked-knee toe touches can strain the knees and pull the hamstring muscles in the thigh. The basic rule for stretching is simple: If a movement hurts, stop doing it. (See also AEROBIC DANCE; FITNESS; FITNESS TRAINING; RUNNING.)

▶ SUGAR

Sugar is the simplest type of CARBOHYDRATE, a NUTRIENT that the body needs in large amounts. The other two types of carbohydrate are STARCH and FIBER. A major source of energy, sugar is an important part of the diet.

The U.S. Department of Agriculture estimates that the average person consumes about 43 pounds (19.6 kg) of sugar a year. Although the body needs sugar, there are good reasons to limit its consumption. Many sugary foods are high in FAT and CALORIES and low in PROTEIN, VITAMINS, and MINERALS. Excessive amounts of sugar are easily converted to BODY FAT and can also cause tooth decay.

In chemistry, sugars are known as *saccharides*. Depending on its chemical structure, a sugar is classified either as a *monosaccharide* (one sugar unit) or as a *disaccharide,* two monosaccharide units linked together. The chemical names for sugars always end in *-ose*. Glucose, fructose, sucrose, galactose, lactose, and maltose are the six sugars found in foods.

Types of Sugar   GLUCOSE, also known as *dextrose,* is a monosaccharide. It is highly soluble and moves quickly into the bloodstream (where it is known as blood sugar). Glucose is found in nearly all foods of plant origin.

Fructose is a monosaccharide and the sweetest of all the sugars. Also called fruit sugar, it is found in fruits and saps. A disadvantage of this

Sugar Sources. *The body needs sugar, but not all foods that contain sugar are equally nutritious. A can of soda is little more than sugar and water, but an orange has the additional benefits of vitamins, minerals, and fiber.*

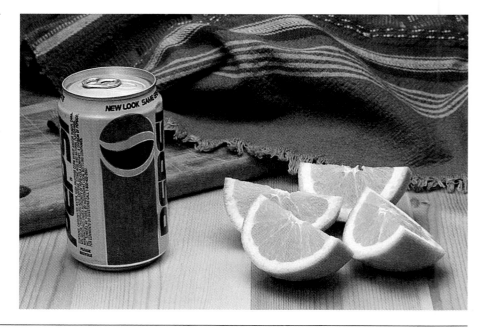

sugar is that it is more readily converted than are other forms of sugar into fat that circulates in the blood.

Sucrose, familiar as table sugar, is the best known of the three disaccharides. Chemically, it is the union of the monosaccharides glucose and fructose. Its principal sources are sugar cane and sugar beets, and it is also found in a number of fruits, vegetables, and grains. The fructose component of sucrose makes this sugar very sweet; it is widely used in candy, soft drinks, and baked goods, among many other foods.

Lactose is a disaccharide that combines glucose and a rarely occurring monosaccharide known as galactose. Lactose is often called milk sugar because it makes up about 5 percent of milk. Babies can easily digest lactose from the moment they are born, which makes milk sugar an excellent source of energy for infants. Some people, however, later develop an inability to digest lactose, a condition known as *lactose intolerance.* This condition becomes more common with age. (See also FOOD ALLERGIES AND INTOLERANCES.)

Forms of Sugar   Sugar comes in many different forms that have distinctive appearances and flavors. For example, sugar cane yields a thick, brown syrup known as *molasses,* which can be mixed with white sugar to produce *brown sugar. Honey* is made by bees from the nectar of flowers, whereas *maple syrup* is made by boiling down the sap of maple trees. Because these sweeteners have a stronger flavor than table sugar, it may be possible to use smaller amounts of them than you would of sugar. However, contrary to popular opinion, none of these sweeteners is more nutritious than table sugar. All of them are disaccharides made up of glucose and fructose and contain no vitamins or minerals. (See also ARTIFICIAL SWEETENERS; ENERGY, FOOD; FATS, OILS, AND SWEETS; OVERWEIGHT; DIABETES, **3.**)

▶ **SWIMMING**

HEALTHY CHOICES
●●●●●●●●●●●●

Swimming is an excellent form of AEROBIC EXERCISE. It improves the efficiency of the heart and lungs and uses nearly every muscle group in the body. Swimming rarely causes injuries because the water supports a swimmer and thus reduces stress on muscles, joints, and bones. All of these factors make swimming a FITNESS exercise of special value for people with disabilities as well as for those recovering from injuries.

Swimming for Fitness   An aerobic swimming workout consists of 30 to 40 minutes of continuous swimming three to four times a week. The best stroke for both burning CALORIES and promoting fitness is the freestyle, or forward crawl. A *length* is the distance from one end of the pool to the other. A *lap* is the distance from one end of the pool to the other and back. People usually begin with a few laps and add more until they are swimming 1 to 1.5 miles (about 1.6 to 2.4 km) at each session. In an Olympic-size swimming pool, 16 laps equals just under 1 mile.

Swimming takes up to four times as much effort as RUNNING to cover an equal distance, so swimmers need to swim only one-fourth as far to expend the same number of calories as runners do. On the other hand, because swimming is not a *weight-bearing exercise,* it may not strengthen

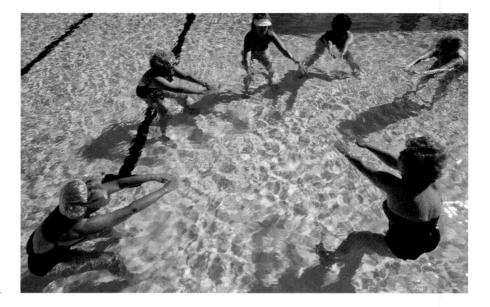

Swimming for Fitness. *Swimming is an excellent overall fitness exercise for many people.*

bones or provide the same protection against osteoporosis as some other sports.

Convenience and Safety Since swimming for exercise requires good basic skills, beginners should take lessons before starting a swimming program. Most swimmers have to locate an indoor pool and travel there to exercise, so swimming may be inconvenient for people with full schedules. In addition, swimmers are prone to dry skin, eye and sinus irritation, and swimmer's ear (a fungal infection of the ear canal). Goggles, ear plugs, nose clips, and special ear drops can prevent some of these problems. For safety, never swim alone; never dive into water unless you know that it is deep enough; and never swim in excessively cold water. Very cold water can cause *hypothermia,* a condition of dangerously low body temperature. (See also EAR INFECTIONS, **2**; HYPOTHERMIA, **8**.)

RISK FACTORS
► ► ► ► ► ►

► **UNDERWEIGHT** People who are more than 15 percent below the recommended weight for their height and sex are considered underweight. Eating habits as well as heredity may cause a person to be underweight. Athletes and other people who EXERCISE heavily may become underweight if they do not balance their increased physical activity with increased caloric intake. When an individual is extremely underweight, either due to an illness or because of an EATING DISORDER such as anorexia or bulimia, medical help is needed.

While being slightly underweight does not present a significant health risk, people who are severely underweight can experience a number of physical problems. Because BODY FAT helps to keep the body warm, people who are underweight may feel cold all the time. An underweight body may also be less able to regulate its temperature through perspiration, so that the risk of heat injury during exercise is increased. Severely underweight women may stop menstruating and may have an increased risk of osteoporosis. These two problems, together with eating disorders, are sometimes referred to as the *"female athlete triad."* People who are underweight because of poor eating habits may also develop other problems due to MALNUTRITION. (See also OSTEOPOROSIS.)

To gain weight, try a WEIGHT-GAIN STRATEGY that will increase the number of CALORIES that you eat. Eating larger quantities of healthful foods and snacking sensibly during the day should stimulate weight gain in most cases. Moderate exercise may also stimulate the appetite and help with muscle development. Weight should be gained gradually; about 1 pound (about 0.5 kg) per week is usually considered safe. (See also WEIGHT ASSESSMENT.)

▶ VEGETABLE GROUP

The vegetable food group is made up of foods that come from the edible parts (whether roots, leaves, shoots, or flesh) of a variety of plants. One of the five major food groups of the FOOD GUIDE PYRAMID, this group includes cabbage, asparagus, and peas, among many others. Vegetables are important sources of NUTRIENTS such as CARBOHYDRATES, VITAMINS, and MINERALS. Most vegetables may be eaten raw or cooked. Certain cooking methods, however, significantly reduce the nutritive value of these foods.

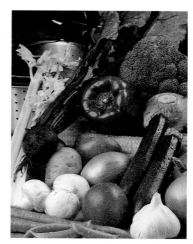

Vegetable Group. *Different vegetables supply varying amounts of nutrients such as carbohydrates, vitamins, minerals, and water.*

Nutrition from Vegetables Vegetables are generally low in CALORIES because much of their weight is made up of WATER. Most vegetables contain little or no FAT, although a few (avocado, for example) are high in fat. There are several different types of vegetables that supply different nutrients.

- *Dark green leafy vegetables,* such as spinach, broccoli, and watercress, are good sources of VITAMIN A and VITAMIN C. They also contain CALCIUM, IRON, and FIBER, a carbohydrate substance that helps move food through the digestive tract.
- *Deep yellow vegetables* include both yellow and orange vegetables, such as carrots, yams, and squash. These vegetables are high in BETA CAROTENE.
- *Starchy vegetables,* including potatoes, corn, and lima beans, contain nearly as much STARCH as foods from the BREAD, CEREAL, RICE, AND PASTA GROUP. They are a part of the vegetable group because they also supply vitamins and minerals found mostly in vegetables, such as POTASSIUM and several parts of the VITAMIN B COMPLEX.
- *Legumes* are seeds that grow in pods, such as chick peas, kidney beans, and black-eyed peas. This type of vegetable is high in PROTEIN and can also be treated as part of the MEAT, POULTRY, DRY BEANS, EGGS, AND NUTS GROUP.

Daily Servings of Vegetables The Food Guide Pyramid recommends that everyone consume three to five servings of vegetables per day. A serving is approximately one-half cup of cooked vegetables, one cup of leafy vegetables, or one small baked potato. Vegetables are best eaten fresh and raw, because they lose vitamin content during storage and cooking. Vegetables are also available frozen or canned. Steaming vegetables or cooking them in small amounts of water retains their nutrients better than boiling or frying. Cooking vegetables in a small amount of water in a

HEALTHY CHOICES
▪▪▪▪▪▪▪▪▪▪▪

microwave oven will also retain most of their nutrients. Many vegetables, including potatoes and squash, can be baked or roasted to prevent a great loss of nutrients. Avoid peeling vegetables such as potatoes and cucumbers, as the edible skins are high in fiber.

Most Americans do not get enough vegetables in their diets. To increase your intake of vegetables, try adding them to other foods, such as sandwiches and pasta dishes. SNACKING on raw vegetables instead of less nutritious snack foods is another good way to add vegetables to your diet. (See also DIETARY GUIDELINES; EXCHANGE SYSTEM; FATS, OILS, AND SWEETS; MILK, YOGURT, AND CHEESE GROUP.)

▶ **VEGETARIAN DIET**   A vegetarian diet is one that includes no meat, poultry, or fish. Vegetarian diets are healthy and nutritious as long as they include a variety of foods that, together, provide adequate amounts of VITAMINS, MINERALS, and PROTEINS as well as enough CALORIES.

Millions of people all over the world are *vegetarians,* or people who eat a vegetarian diet. Some people choose to eat a vegetarian diet for religious, ethical, or health-related reasons. In many developing countries, however, people may be vegetarians out of necessity because they cannot afford to raise or buy meat.

Types of Vegetarians   There are several different types of vegetarians. *Vegans,* or strict vegetarians, will not consume any animal products; they eat only vegetables, fruits, nuts, and grains. *Lactovegetarians* add milk products to their diet, whereas *lacto-ovovegetarians* include both milk products and eggs. *Semivegetarians* eat milk products, eggs, and an occasional serving of fish or poultry.

In addition to these four basic types of vegetarian diets, there are several more specialized types. For example, a *whole-food diet* includes only foods in their natural form, with none of the edible parts removed. A *fruitarian* diet is made up entirely of plant foods that can be harvested without killing the plant. A *macrobiotic* diet, based on the Eastern philosophy of balanced yin and yang (male and female energy), may include few or no animal products; the strictest macrobiotic diets consist only of brown rice and teas. Some people believe that a macrobiotic diet can cure cancer by cleansing the body of *toxins* (harmful substances). There is no scientific evidence that it does so, however. In fact, strict macrobiotic diets can damage the body through MALNUTRITION. (See also FAD DIETS.)

Eating a Balanced Diet   Vegetarians, especially vegans, must be careful to eat a varied, well-balanced diet in adequate amounts. Certain essential NUTRIENTS are much more common in meats, milk products, and eggs than in foods of plant origin. Vegetarians must therefore adjust their diets to provide all the vitamins, minerals, and protein their bodies need.

One such vitamin is *vitamin B_{12},* which is found mostly in animal products such as meat, liver, eggs, and milk. A lack of vitamin B_{12} can cause permanent damage to the brain and nerves, so it is especially dangerous to developing infants and children. Vegans can obtain vitamin B_{12}

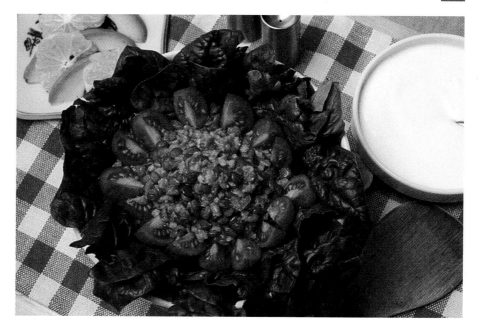

Eating a Vegetarian Diet. *People who eat a vegetarian diet must eat a variety of foods to obtain all the nutrients their bodies need.*

from a vitamin supplement or from foods that have been fortified with vitamin B_{12}. A few plant foods, such as nutritional yeast and wheat germ, contain small amounts of this vitamin.

Also lacking in most vegan diets is VITAMIN D, which is found primarily in fish oils, beef, butter, eggs, and fortified milk. This vitamin is essential for normal bone and tooth development. Because plant foods are not a source of vitamin D, vegans must either take a vitamin D supplement or be sure to get regular exposure to the sun, which prompts the body to manufacture its own supply of the vitamin.

A deficiency of IRON, an important nutrient, may also be a problem for vegetarians. Although present in many vegetables and grains, iron is more easily absorbed from animal products such as meat and poultry. Vegetarians who do not eat animal products should eat plant foods that are high in iron, such as dried beans, spinach, dried fruits, and tofu.

Lactovegetarians and lacto-ovovegetarians can get plenty of CALCIUM from dairy products. Although many foods of plant origin contain calcium as well, they must usually be consumed in large quantities to provide the amount found in milk and dairy products. Vegans (especially infants and children, who require more calcium for healthy development) may need supplements or calcium-fortified soy products, cereal, and orange juice as a part of their diet.

All vegetarians must ensure that they eat an adequate amount of protein. This may be especially difficult for vegans, because most plant proteins are incomplete; they do not contain all of the essential *amino acids*. As a result, vegans need to consume proteins from different plant sources throughout the day in order to supply themselves with complete proteins. In general, the amino acids from grains (such as rice) form complete proteins when combined with the amino acids from legumes (such as kidney beans). The foods need not be eaten at the same meal to allow the proteins to combine. There are also a few plant foods—soybeans, dried yeast, and wheat germ—that do provide complete proteins.

HEALTHY CHOICES
●●●●●●●●●●●●

HEALTHY CHOICES
●●●●●●●●●●●●●

Benefits of a Vegetarian Diet   When adequate in amount and variety, vegetarian diets offer significant health benefits. They are usually lower in FATS and higher in FIBER than diets that include meat, so they lower the likelihood of colon cancer and diverticulitis while aiding in weight loss. Studies have shown that a low-fat vegetarian diet reduces the risks of heart disease and diabetes. In addition, vegan diets are free of CHOLESTEROL, low in saturated fats (which serves to lower blood cholesterol levels), low in SODIUM, and high in POTASSIUM (which reduces the risk of hypertension). However, not all vegetarian foods are low in fat, so vegetarians, like other people, must be careful to avoid too much fat and eat plenty of vitamin-rich fruits, vegetables, and whole grains. (See also DIETARY GUIDELINES; DIETS; NUTRITION; VITAMIN B COMPLEX.)

► VITAMIN A

Vitamin A is an organic chemical substance that is essential to normal growth and the development of strong bones and teeth. Also called *retinol,* it promotes healthy cell structure in the skin and in the linings of the respiratory, digestive, and urinary tracts, which protect these systems from infection. Vitamin A also promotes normal vision. The body can get vitamin A from foods or manufacture it from BETA CAROTENE, one of the PHYTOCHEMICALS found in many vegetables and fruits.

Prescription medications have recently been developed from vitamin A. These medications are applied directly to the skin to treat acne and the skin damage that results from too much sun exposure.

Sampling of Foods Rich in Vitamin A. *The recommended dietary allowance for vitamin A is 1,000 mcg for men and 800 mcg for women. Foods rich in this vitamin include beef liver, carrots, and winter squash.*

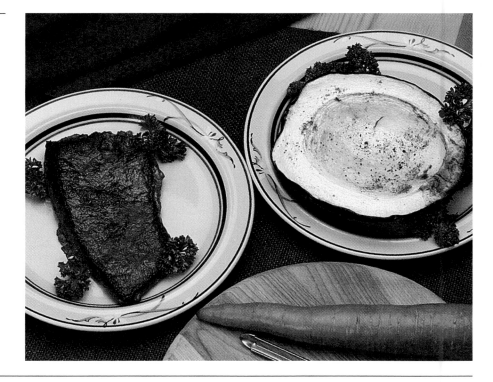

Vitamin A Deficiency   A deficiency of vitamin A is rare in a developed country like the United States, but it can result from vitamin absorption problems in the intestine or from long-term treatment with certain drugs. Poor diets in developing countries, however, result in vitamin A deficiencies in many children. Symptoms of deficiency include dry, inflamed eyes, poor night vision, or blindness; dry, rough skin; loss of appetite; diarrhea; lowered resistance to infection; and, in severe cases, weak bones and teeth.

RISK FACTORS
▶ ▶ ▶ ▶ ▶ ▶

Recommended Intake of Vitamin A   Vitamin A is a *fat-soluble vitamin.* The RECOMMENDED DIETARY ALLOWANCE (RDA) for vitamin A is 1,000 mcg for men and 800 mcg for women. It is stored in the body's liver and fatty tissue, which can hold up to a year's supply. However, excessive amounts can build up, leading to symptoms such as headache, tiredness, nausea, loss of appetite, diarrhea, weight loss, dry and itchy skin, and hair loss. In women, too much vitamin A can cause irregular menstrual periods and, if consumed during pregnancy, birth defects. Extreme cases of excess vitamin A may cause swollen feet and ankles, bone pain, and enlargement of the liver and spleen.

HEALTHY CHOICES
■●●●●●●●●●●●■

Sources of Vitamin A   Rich sources of vitamin A include liver, fish-liver oils, egg yolk, milk and dairy products, and margarine. Good sources of beta carotene include carrots, sweet potatoes, winter squash, kale, broccoli, spinach, apricots, and peaches. (See also VITAMINS.)

▶ VITAMIN B COMPLEX

Vitamin B complex is a group of vitamins that includes *thiamine* (vitamin B_1), *riboflavin* (B_2), *niacin, pantothenic acid, pyridoxine* (B_6), *biotin, folate,* and *vitamin B_{12}* (cobalamin). As a group, these vitamins are essential to energy metabolism and health maintenance. Each component of this complex of vitamins is important to good health. Harmful effects from excess doses of B vitamins are rare because these vitamins are *water-soluble,* so the body normally excretes what it does not use. Animal products are good sources of most B vitamins, as are whole grains (see chart: Foods Rich in B Complex Vitamins). Processed grain products, such as white bread, may lack B vitamins unless the products are *enriched,* meaning that lost nutrients have been replaced after processing. Women who are pregnant or breast-feeding need greater amounts of all the B vitamins.

Thiamine   Thiamine aids enzymes (substances that produce chemical reactions) in breaking down and using carbohydrates. It also helps the nerves, muscles, and heart to function efficiently. A mild deficiency causes tiredness, irritability, loss of appetite, and sleeping problems. A severe deficiency can cause beriberi (a disease affecting the nerves in the legs), abdominal pain, depression, constipation, and impaired memory. Elderly people who eat a poor diet, people with extremely high energy requirements, or people with overactive thyroid glands may experience thiamine deficiency. For most people, however, a varied diet provides enough of this vitamin. The RECOMMENDED DIETARY ALLOWANCE (RDA) for thiamine is 1.2 mg for men and 1.1 mg for women.

RISK FACTORS
▶ ▶ ▶ ▶ ▶ ▶

FOODS RICH IN B COMPLEX VITAMINS	
Vitamin	**Foods**
Thiamine	Whole-grain breads and cereals, wheat germ, bran, brown rice, pasta, legumes, eggs, fish, pork, liver
Riboflavin	Liver, milk, eggs, cheese, whole-grain and enriched breads and cereals, brewer's yeast, leafy green vegetables
Niacin	Liver, lean meat, poultry, fish, whole grains, nuts, dried beans
Pantothenic acid, pyroxidine, biotin	Meats, fish, whole grains, wheat germ, potatoes, dried beans, fruits, vegetables
Folate	Leafy green vegetables, dried beans, wheat germ, fruits, fortified grain products
Vitamin B_{12}	Fish, meat, milk, poultry, eggs

Riboflavin Riboflavin helps the enzymes that break down carbohydrates, fats, and proteins and convert them to energy. A deficiency may cause chapped lips, soreness in and around the mouth, and eye disorders. The RDA for riboflavin is 1.3 mg for men and 1.1 mg for women.

Niacin Niacin helps enzymes break down carbohydrates and fats, maintains nervous and digestive systems, helps glands produce sex hormones, and promotes healthy skin. Niacin in large doses is sometimes prescribed by doctors to treat high blood cholesterol levels. A deficiency can cause sore and cracked skin, mouth and tongue inflammation, and mental disturbances. The body can get niacin from food or manufacture it from the amino acid *tryptophan*, so the RDA for niacin is given in *niacin equivalents* (NE): 16 mg NE for men and 14 mg NE for women.

RISK FACTORS
▶ ▶ ▶ ▶ ▶ ▶

Pantothenic Acid, Pyridoxine (B$_6$), and Biotin These vitamins aid enzymes that break down carbohydrates, fats, and proteins. Deficiencies are rare among people who eat a varied diet. Extremely high amounts of pyridoxine are believed to cause a problem with the nervous system called neuritis. The RDA for pyroxidine is 1.3 mg daily for men through age 50 and 1.7 mg daily thereafter, 1.2 mg for girls from age 14 to 18, 1.3 mg for women through age 50, and 1.5 mg daily thereafter. No RDA exists for biotin or pantothenic acid, although *adequate intakes* have been established.

Folate and Vitamin B$_{12}$ Vitamin B_{12} and folate work together to produce red blood cells. Vitamin B_{12} helps the body use amino acids and fatty acids, and folate assists in producing DNA, the part of cells that stores the body's hereditary characteristics. *Folic acid*, a synthetic form of folate, is added to all enriched grain products such as flour, pasta, and cereal. A deficiency of either vitamin produces *anemia*, a deficiency of red blood cells. Insufficient amounts of folate during pregnancy are linked to an increased risk of certain birth defects, such as spina bifida. Adults should consume 2.4 mcg of vitamin B_{12} daily. Both men and women need 400 mcg of folate each day. (See also VEGETARIAN DIET; VITAMINS; ANEMIA, **3**.)

RISK FACTORS
▶ ▶ ▶ ▶ ▶ ▶

► VITAMIN C

Vitamin C is an organic chemical substance that performs several important functions. Also called *ascorbic acid,* it works with enzymes (substances that spark chemical reactions in the body) to develop and maintain healthy bones, teeth, gums, ligaments, and blood vessels. Vitamin C helps produce chemicals that transmit nerve impulses and adrenal gland hormones. It also helps the body heal its wounds and absorb iron from the digestive tract.

Studies have suggested that vitamin C may play a role in preventing cancer, slowing the development of heart disease, and helping the immune system fight infection. This may be due to the vitamin's *antioxidant* properties. Vitamins that are antioxidants are able to fight certain chemical substances called *free radicals* that damage cells, opening the door for disease and the effects of aging. (See also VITAMIN E.)

RISK FACTORS
► ► ► ► ► ►

Vitamin C Deficiency   A mild deficiency of vitamin C can cause swollen gums, nosebleeds, and general aches and pains. Severe deficiency can lead to *anemia,* a deficiency of red blood cells, or *scurvy,* a rare and potentially fatal disease.

Recommended Intake of Vitamin C   Vitamin C is a *water-soluble vitamin,* so it cannot be stored in large amounts in the body. A regular supply must be included in the diet. The RECOMMENDED DIETARY ALLOWANCE (RDA) for vitamin C for people 15 years and older is 60 mg, an amount usually included in a balanced diet. Some scientists believe that very high doses of vitamin C can prevent colds, but the evidence is inconclusive. Furthermore, large doses may cause nausea, stomach cramps, diarrhea, and kidney stones.

HEALTHY CHOICES
• • • • • • • • • • • •

Sources of Vitamin C   Vitamin C is found in fresh fruits and vegetables. Citrus fruits, tomatoes, leafy green vegetables, potatoes, green peppers, strawberries, and cantaloupe are excellent sources. Vitamin C is more effective when accompanied by *bioflavonoids,* substances that occur naturally in fruits and vegetables and that complement vitamin C. Foods rich

Sampling of Foods Rich in Vitamin C.   *The recommended dietary allowance for vitamin C is 60 mg per day. Foods rich in this vitamin include oranges, broccoli, and cantaloupe.*

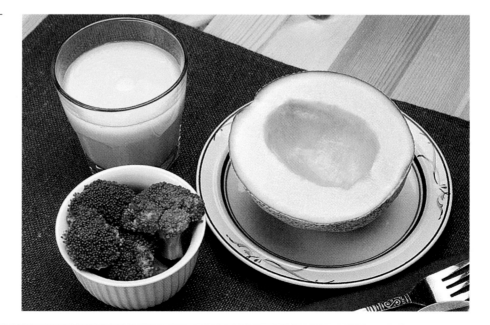

in both elements include citrus fruits, cherries, rose hips, sweet and hot peppers, spinach, and other dark green leafy vegetables. (See also VITAMINS; ANEMIA, **3**.)

▶ VITAMIN D

Vitamin D is a group of related organic chemical substances that, together, maintain strong bones and teeth by controlling the body's use of CALCIUM and phosphorus. Vitamin D helps regulate levels of calcium and phosphate in the bones and blood and stimulates the kidneys to retain calcium. Besides being present in many foods, vitamin D is also produced by the body when the skin is exposed to sunlight. It is a *fat-soluble vitamin* that is stored in the body's fatty tissue and in the liver. Fortified milk and other dairy products, oily fish, liver, and egg yolks are rich sources of vitamin D.

RISK FACTORS
▶ ▶ ▶ ▶ ▶ ▶

Recommended Intake of Vitamin D   Either too little or too much vitamin D can cause medical problems. The *adequate intake* for vitamin D is 5 mcg for children and adults through age 50. From age 51 to 70, the adequate intake is 10 mcg, and it is 15 mcg for people over age 70. Excess vitamin D in the body is rarely caused by eating too many foods with high levels of the vitamin. Large doses of vitamin D supplements, however, can cause weakness, abnormal thirst, increased urination, gastrointestinal disturbances, and depression. Because vitamin D is fat soluble, excessive intake over a long period can cause calcium deposits in the kidneys and hardening of blood vessel walls. (See also RECOMMENDED DIETARY ALLOWANCE.)

RISK FACTORS
▶ ▶ ▶ ▶ ▶ ▶

Vitamin D Deficiency   Vitamin D deficiency can lead to a softening of the bones. In children, this condition is called *rickets;* in adults, it is called *osteomalacia.* Deficiencies are rare but can occur among people who eat a poor diet; who have a disorder that prevents the intestine from

Sampling of Foods Rich in Vitamin D. *The adequate intake of vitamin D is between 5 and 15 mcg per day, depending on age. Foods rich in this vitamin include eggs, liver, fortified milk, tuna, salmon, and sardines.*

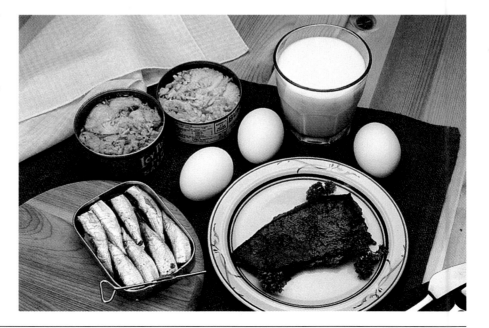

absorbing the vitamin; or who are deprived of sunlight for some reason, such as working at night. (See also VITAMINS.)

▶ VITAMIN E

Vitamin E, a group of organic chemical substances, performs a number of vital functions. It is essential for creating and sustaining normal cell structure, forming red blood cells, and maintaining the activity of enzymes (substances that promote chemical reactions in the body). In addition, vitamin E is an *antioxidant*, which means that it is able to fight certain molecules called *free radicals* that damage red blood cells and lung tissue, opening the door for disease. A lack of vitamin E leads to destruction of red blood cells and thus causes *anemia.* Vitamin E deficiency is rare and is usually caused by intestinal absorption problems or liver disorders.

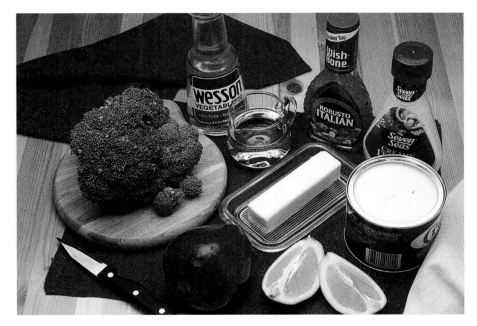

Sampling of Foods Rich in Vitamin E. *The recommended dietary allowance for most adults for vitamin E is 8 to 10 mg per day. Foods rich in this vitamin include many fruits, vegetables, and vegetable oil products, such as margarine, salad dressings, shortening, soybean oils, and wheat germ oil.*

Vitamin E is a *fat-soluble vitamin,* which means that it is stored for long periods in the liver and fatty tissues. The RECOMMENDED DIETARY ALLOWANCE (RDA) for vitamin E is 8 mg for females age 11 and over; it is 10 mg for men age 11 and over as well as for pregnant women. Breast-feeding women need 11 to 12 mg daily. Excessive intake of vitamin E may cause abdominal pain, nausea, and diarrhea.

A balanced diet provides adequate vitamin E, which is found in large amounts in vegetable oils, nuts, meats, leafy green vegetables, cereals, wheat germ, and egg yolks. (See also VITAMIN C; VITAMINS.)

▶ VITAMIN K

Vitamin K is a group of organic chemical substances that are essential for blood clotting. A *fat-soluble vitamin,* vitamin K is stored in the liver and fatty tissues. Rich sources of vitamin K include leafy green vegetables,

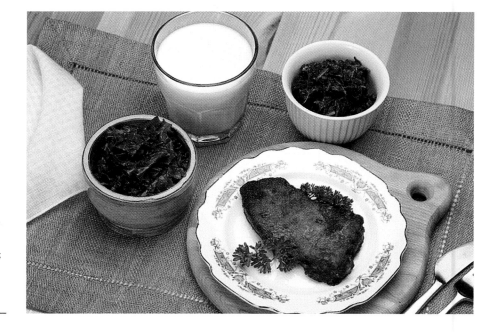

Sampling of Foods Rich in Vitamin K. *The recommended dietary allowance for vitamin K is 60 to 80 mcg for adults. Foods rich in this vitamin include spinach, kale, milk, pork, and liver.*

RISK FACTORS
▶ ▶ ▶ ▶ ▶ ▶

cauliflower, vegetable oils, egg yolks, cheese, pork, and liver. A deficiency of vitamin K reduces the blood's ability to clot and may result in abnormal bleeding from the nose, gums, intestines, or urinary tract.

Deficiencies of vitamin K are rare because it is readily available in the diet and is also produced by intestinal bacteria. Supplements of vitamin K are given to newborns, however, because they do not have enough intestinal bacteria to produce vitamin K until they are about 2 weeks old.

The RECOMMENDED DIETARY ALLOWANCE (RDA) of vitamin K is 45 to 65 mcg for teenagers and 60 to 80 mcg for adults. Daily intake above this level has no known harmful effects. (See also VITAMINS.)

▶ VITAMINS

Vitamins are organic chemical substances that trigger a wide variety of bodily processes. Essential to human health, they are required in very small amounts that are generally supplied by a balanced diet. A few are manufactured by the body itself. The 13 known vitamins are A, C, D, E, K, and the 8 vitamins that make up the B-complex.

Vitamins are divided into two groups: fat-soluble vitamins (A, D, E, and K) and water-soluble vitamins (C and B complex vitamins). *Fat-soluble vitamins* can be stored in the liver and fatty tissues. *Water-soluble vitamins* are stored in the body for only a short time, and any excess passes out of the body in urine.

HEALTHY CHOICES
● ● ● ● ● ● ● ● ● ● ● ●

Currently, the RECOMMENDED DIETARY ALLOWANCES (RDAs) provide guidelines for meeting most people's daily needs for some vitamins and avoiding deficiency or toxicity (see chart: Recommended Dietary Allowances for Four Vitamins). However, the Food and Nutrition Board of the National Academy of Sciences is in the process of creating new recommendations, *dietary reference intakes* (DRIs), to update the RDAs (see chart: Dietary Reference Intakes [DRIs] for Vitamin B Complex and

RECOMMENDED DIETARY ALLOWANCES FOR FOUR VITAMINS

Category (age, sex, or condition)	Vitamin A (*)	Vitamin E (mg)	Vitamin K (mcg)	Vitamin C (mg)
Infants				
0–1/2	375	3	5	30
1/2–1	375	4	10	35
Children				
1–3	400	6	15	40
4–6	500	7	20	45
7–10	700	7	30	45
Males				
11–14	1,000	10	45	50
15–18	1,000	10	65	60
19–24	1,000	10	70	60
25–50	1,000	10	80	60
51+	1,000	10	80	60
Females				
11–14	800	8	45	50
15–18	800	8	55	60
19–24	800	8	60	60
25–50	800	8	65	60
51+	800	8	65	60
Pregnant females	800	10	65	70
Lactating females				
1st 6 months	1,300	12	65	95
2nd 6 months	1,200	11	65	90

*Mcg RE (retinol equivalent). 1 RE is equal to 1 mcg of retinol or 6 mcg of beta carotene.
Source: Reprinted with permission from *Recommended Dietary Allowances, 10th ed.* Copyright © 1989 by National Academy Press, Washington, D.C.

Vitamin D). A healthful, varied diet usually provides all the vitamins a person needs. Vitamin deficiency diseases, therefore, are rare in the United States. Certain circumstances, however, can increase the body's need for vitamins: for example, some illnesses, pregnancy, and breast-feeding. In these situations, a doctor may prescribe vitamin supplements.

Emerging research suggests that ingesting certain vitamins in doses above the RDA guidelines can protect against some diseases, including heart disease and cancer, and some effects of aging, such as cataracts. But many medical experts believe that the information is too new to include in updated recommendations to the general public. In particular, questions involving amounts of vitamins and the form in which they should be taken are currently unresolved. "Megadoses," or very large doses, are known to cause a dangerous excess of some vitamins. An excess of

RISK FACTORS
▶ ▶ ▶ ▶ ▶ ▶

DIETARY REFERENCE INTAKES (DRIS) FOR VITAMIN B COMPLEX AND VITAMIN D

Age/Life Stage	Thiamine (mg)	Riboflavin (mg)	Niacin[a] (mg)	Vitamin B$_6$ (mg)	Folate[b] (mcg)	Vitamin B$_{12}$ (mcg)	Pantothenic Acid (mg)	Biotin (mcg)	Vitamin D[d,e] (mcg)
Infants									
0–5 months	0.2*	0.3*	2*	0.1*	65*	0.4*	1.7*	5*	5*
6–11 months	0.3*	0.4*	3*	0.3*	80*	0.5*	1.8*	6*	5*
Children									
1–3 years	0.5	0.5	6	0.5	150	0.9	2*	8*	5*
4–8 years	0.6	0.6	8	0.6	200	1.2	3*	12*	5*
Males									
9–13 years	0.9	0.9	12	1.0	300	1.8	4*	20*	5*
14–18 years	1.2	1.3	16	1.3	400	2.4	5*	25*	5*
19–30 years	1.2	1.3	16	1.3	400	2.4	5*	30*	5*
31–50 years	1.2	1.3	16	1.3	400	2.4	5*	30*	5*
51–70 years	1.2	1.3	16	1.7	400	2.4c	5*	30*	10*
>70 years	1.2	1.3	16	1.7	400	2.4c	5*	30*	15*
Females									
9–13 years	0.9	0.9	12	1.0	300	1.8	4*	20*	5*
14–18 years	1.0	1.0	14	1.2	400	2.4	5*	25*	5*
19–30 years	1.1	1.1	14	1.3	400	2.4	5*	30*	5*
31–50 years	1.1	1.1	14	1.5	400	2.4	5*	30*	5*
51–70 years	1.1	1.1	14	1.5	400	2.4c	5*	30*	10*
>70 years	1.1	1.1	14	1.5	400	2.4c	5*	30*	15*
Pregnancy									
≤18 years	1.4	1.4	18	1.9	600	2.6	6*	30*	5*
19–30 years	1.4	1.4	18	1.9	600	2.6	6*	30*	5*
31–50 years	1.4	1.4	18	1.9	600	2.6	6*	30*	5*
Lactation									
≤18 years	1.5	1.6	17	2.0	500	2.8	7*	35*	5*
19–30 years	1.5	1.6	17	2.0	500	2.8	7*	35*	5*
31–50 years	1.5	1.6	17	2.0	500	2.8	7*	35*	5*

*Note: This table presents Recommended Dietary Allowances (RDAs) and Adequate Intakes (AIs). AI values are followed by an asterisk.

[a]As niacin equivalents. 1 mg of niacin = 60 mg of tryptophan.

[b]As dietary folate equivalents (DFE). 1 DFE = 1 mcg food folate = 0.6 mcg of folic acid (from fortified food or supplement) consumed with food = 0.5 mcg of supplemental folic acid taken on an empty stomach.

[c]Since 10 to 30 percent of older people may malabsorb food-bound B$_{12}$, it is advisable for people over age 50 to meet their RDA mainly by eating foods fortified with B$_{12}$ or a supplement containing B$_{12}$.

[d]As cholecalciferol (1 mcg cholecalciferol = 40 IU vitamin D).

[e]In the absence of adequate exposure to sunlight.

Source: Reprinted with permission from Dietary Reference Intakes (prepublication versions). In press, National Academy Press. Courtesy of National Academy Press, Washington, D.C.

fat-soluble vitamins is especially harmful. These vitamins build up in the fatty tissues in the body and can reach toxic levels. Traditional medical opinion holds that taking vitamin supplements in doses within the RDA guidelines has no negative health effects but also offers but no significant health benefits other than to help prevent deficiency diseases such as rickets. (See also VITAMIN A; VITAMIN B COMPLEX; VITAMIN C; VITAMIN D; VITAMIN E; VITAMIN K.)

▶ WALKING

Walking is a good exercise to strengthen the heart and lungs, improve overall FITNESS, and maintain or reduce weight. People of any age and virtually any fitness level can walk for exercise. It can be done year-round and requires no special equipment except for a pair of comfortable, well-made walking shoes.

HEALTHY CHOICES
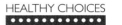

Benefits of Walking Walking for EXERCISE offers many benefits. In addition to strengthening the heart and lungs, it helps reduce blood pressure and blood CHOLESTEROL levels. It tones and strengthens muscles and improves circulation. Because walking is a weight-bearing exercise, it also strengthens bones and reduces the risk of later developing *osteoporosis*, a disease that causes bones to become brittle and more likely to fracture, especially in women.

Like RUNNING, SWIMMING, and CYCLING, walking is an AEROBIC EXERCISE. It elevates the HEART RATE and increases the ability of the body to use oxygen. Walking burns almost as many calories as running the same distance, but it requires less effort and causes fewer injuries. A 160-pound (about 72-kg) person who walks briskly—at a rate of about 3.5 miles (just under 6 km) per hour—for 30 minutes can burn more than 150 calories.

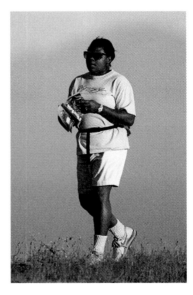

Walking for Fitness. *Walking alone or with friends can be a very pleasant way to exercise.*

Walking Strategies Walking for exercise is different from casual walking or strolling. To walk for exercise, walk in a smooth, steady rhythm as you swing your arms briskly. With each step, land on your heel and push off with the toe. Carrying hand weights of up to 3 pounds (about 1.4 kg) gives the upper body a workout and increases the aerobic effect.

To begin a walking program, start out by walking for 20 to 25 minutes, three times a week. Gradually increase the pace and frequency of your walks until you can walk briskly for 30 to 60 minutes five times a week. Some people walk measured miles; others walk for specific lengths of time. The most important part of any program is that it be a regular part of a weekly routine.

Walking Safety Walking seldom causes injuries, but out-of-shape walkers may experience soreness in the hips and shins. Warm-up exercises that stretch and flex the hip and leg muscles can minimize soreness. Do not stop walking abruptly; allow a cooldown period to prevent your muscles from tightening. Wear loose, comfortable clothing, and dress warmly in winter to avoid losing body heat. Many enclosed shopping malls have walking programs that allow people to exercise safely in any kind of weather. (See also ATHLETIC FOOTWEAR; ENDURANCE.)

▶ WARM-UP AND COOLDOWN

Warm-up and cooldown are the exercises and activities performed before and after engaging in a sport or other physical activity. The purpose of warming up is to prepare the body for EXERCISE. The purpose of cooling down is to ease the body's transition from vigorous activity back to its normal state. Warm-ups and

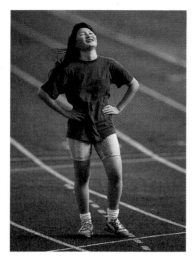

Warm-up and Cooldown.
Warm-up exercises warm your muscles and make them more flexible. Cooldown routines help your body return to its resting

cooldowns are both essential, although often neglected, components of an exercise routine.

Warming Up   The purpose of warming up is literally to raise the temperature of the muscles. Warm muscles are more supple and better protected against pulls, strains, and tears. The most effective warm-up is one that uses the same muscles that will be involved in the actual physical activity. For example, before running 3 miles, a runner might jog gently for several minutes. The longer and more intense the intended physical activity, the longer the warm-up should be.

The warm-up should be followed by gentle STRETCHING EXERCISE. Stretching lengthens the muscles and tendons, improving FLEXIBILITY. Stretched muscles are less likely to tear during exercise.

Cooling Down   After a period of physical activity, a cooldown helps the body return to its resting state. If a person abruptly stops physical activity, blood tends to collect in the lower body. If enough blood does not reach the brain, the person may feel dizzy. Cooling down gradually helps prevent such dizziness and also reduces the likelihood of muscle stiffness. The best approach to cooling down is to repeat the warm-up: a few minutes or more of easy exercise followed by gentle stretching.

▶ WATER

Water is the most abundant substance in the human body, accounting for 55 to 70 percent of the average adult's weight. One of the six basic NUTRIENTS, it is present in and vital to the operation of every living cell and tissue.

Water is essential to life: Without it, humans can survive for only a few days. For that reason, the body maintains a careful balance between water consumed (in foods and beverages) and water lost (through urination, perspiration, and respiration).

Functions of Water   One of the chief functions of water in the body is to carry dissolved nutrients to the cells. This is done by both the *blood* and the *lymph* (a fluid that bathes all soft tissue); both consist largely of water. These fluids also carry away the cells' waste products. The *kidneys* then filter out these wastes and pass them out of the body in the form of *urine,* which is also composed largely of water. (See also URINARY TRACT, 1.)

Water performs a number of additional functions in the body. Among them is its role in physically breaking down foods to aid in DIGESTION. It also acts as a *catalyst* in many chemical reactions. Water in the form of perspiration cools the body through the process of evaporation. Water is also the main ingredient of body fluids that cushion and protect vital organs, including the brain and various organs in the abdomen.

HEALTHY CHOICES

Water in the Diet   Most healthy individuals should consume the equivalent of 8 to 12 glasses of water a day, depending on the weather and their level of physical activity. Most of this water usually comes from BEVERAGES such as tap water, coffee, tea, milk, fruit juices, and soft drinks. The remainder of the body's intake of water comes from solid foods. Fruits and vegetables have a particularly high water content (see illustration: Foods with High Water Content).

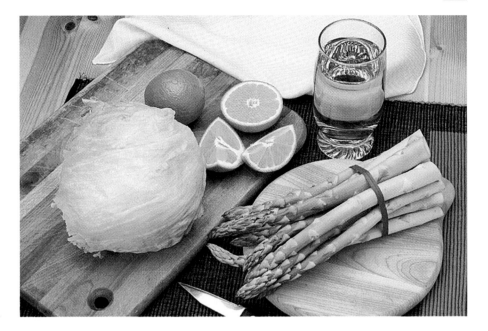

Foods with High Water Content. *One-third of the recommended daily intake of water can come from foods. Foods high in water include lettuce, asparagus, oranges, and potatoes.*

Maintaining a Balance An adequate level of water in the body, called the body's water balance, is maintained by the activities of the kidneys and by changes in *thirst* sensations and fluid intake. When fluid intake is high, the body excretes large quantities of urine. When fluid intake is low, less urine is produced, and more water is absorbed into the blood.

The thirst sensation is triggered by a complex biochemical process that occurs when the body needs more water. Thirst is a person's feeling of a physical need to consume fluids. Food substances such as SUGAR and SALT, which require water to be dissolved, also tend to make a person feel thirsty. The thirst sensation, however, is often a poor guide for adequate fluid intake. People who exercise strenuously or who work in hot climates should drink plenty of fluids even when they are not aware of being thirsty. (See also EXERCISE AND HEAT INJURY.)

RISK FACTORS
▶ ▶ ▶ ▶ ▶ ▶

Too little water in the body can lead to a potentially life-threatening medical condition called DEHYDRATION. This can result from inadequate water intake, excessive water loss, or a combination of the two. Common causes of dehydration include excessive perspiration, due to hot weather or extreme exertion, as well as *diarrhea* and *vomiting*.

In some medical disorders, such as kidney or heart disease, the body cannot excrete excess water adequately. This leads to an accumulation of fluids in the body tissues, a swelling condition called *edema*. (See also BODY METABOLISM; MINERALS; DIURETIC, 7.)

▶ **WEIGHT ASSESSMENT** Weight assessment is the analysis of a person's weight and body composition. BODY COMPOSITION is the ratio of body fat to bone and muscle. Information about your weight and body composition can tell you whether you are UNDERWEIGHT, of normal weight, OVERWEIGHT, or obese. Even if your weight is appropriate, information about body composition can provide one measure of overall FITNESS. Weight assessment

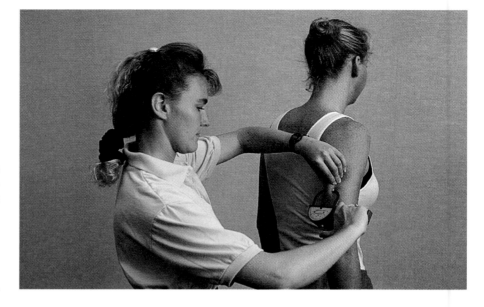

Skinfold Measurement. *To take a skinfold measurement, a health-care professional uses a caliper to measure the amount of fat in a fold of skin at one or more points on the body. Each measurement should be checked two or three times.*

can be used to plan a diet and exercise program that will lead to a positive *body image.*

There are several methods of weight assessment. Some methods compare a person's weight with average weights for men or women of the same height. These methods are convenient, but other, more complex methods are more precise. These methods specifically measure BODY FAT to determine body composition. This is useful because two people of the same height and weight can have different proportions of body fat. One may be out of shape and need to lose some fat, whereas the other's weight may be largely made up of muscle, an indication of fitness.

Assessing Your Own Weight There are several tools available for learning about your own weight. The simplest is a height and weight chart (see chart: Healthy Weight Ranges for Men and Women). Such charts show a range of average weights for each height. People who weigh more than 10 percent above their recommended weight for their height are considered overweight; people more than 20 percent over their recommended weight are considered obese. The advantages of using a chart are its convenience and the ready comparison with averages that it provides. However, charts do not take differences of body type into account.

BODY MASS INDEX (BMI) uses height and weight data in a similar way. Your BMI is a ratio in which weight (in kilograms) is divided by height (in meters) squared. A BMI over 25 indicates that a person is probably overweight. Because excess weight may be muscle rather than fat, however, body mass index should usually be considered together with waist measurement and *waist-to-hip ratio.* This is determined by dividing waist measurement (at the navel) by hip measurement (at the hipbone). For women, the result should be 0.8 or less; for men, 1.0 or less. This method is particularly useful because it measures abdominal fat, which is a greater RISK FACTOR for health problems than is fat in other places in the body.

Assessment by a Health Professional The above methods for assessing weight are simple, but they are not very precise ways of measuring

HEALTHY WEIGHT RANGES FOR MEN AND WOMEN

Height	Weight (in pounds)
4'10"	91–119
4'11"	94–124
5'0"	97–128
5'1"	101–132
5'2"	104–137
5'3"	107–141
5'4"	111–146
5'5"	114–150
5'6"	118–155
5'7"	121–160
5'8"	125–164
5'9"	129–169
5'10"	132–174
5'11"	136–179
6'0"	140–184
6'1"	144–189
6'2"	148–195
6'3"	152–200

body composition. Other tests, performed by a doctor or other health professional, can determine body composition more accurately. A *skinfold measurement* gauges the fat under the skin. An instrument called a caliper is used to measure the thickness of a fold of skin on the back of the upper arm, the shoulder blade, the thigh, or some other area (see illustration: Skinfold Measurement). The measurements are used to estimate body fat. The accuracy of this method depends on the precise use of the caliper. Human error may cause the measurement to vary by as much as 4 percent.

Hydrostatic (or underwater) *weighing* is another method of measuring body fat. Because muscle and bone are heavier and more dense than fat, fat causes the body to float in water. Hydrostatic weighing involves first weighing the person on a regular scale. Then the person is weighed again while he or she is completely submerged in water. The two weight measurements are compared to calculate the amount of fat and lean tissue. Although this is the most accurate method of weight assessment, it is relatively expensive, and some people dislike being under water. A newer test that does not require submersion is nearly as accurate but is not yet in wide use.

The electric conductivity method (also called *bioelectrical impedance*) uses the body's water content to estimate the proportion of fat. Lean tissue contains water, but fat does not. Water will conduct an electric current. In this method, electrodes are attached to a person's wrist and ankles and a weak electric current is sent through the body. A computer notes how much of the current is lost; from this information, the percentage of body fat can be estimated. However, this estimate can be highly inaccurate, especially if the person's body is especially high or low on water when the test is performed.

Uses of Weight Assessment Data Choosing a method of weight assessment in any particular situation depends on the intended purpose. Because a person's mental image of his or her body is often inaccurate, it can be helpful to have an objective assessment before setting weight-change goals. Accurate information about body composition can also help people to learn about their bodies and to focus on those areas that need change. People who are tempted to diet to lose weight sometimes discover that their weight falls within the normal range for their height. Careful weight assessment can save some people the trouble of unnecessary dieting and help others to choose the best diet to meet their needs. (See also DIETS; EATING DISORDERS; WEIGHT-GAIN STRATEGY; WEIGHT-LOSS STRATEGY.)

HEALTHY CHOICES

► WEIGHT-GAIN STRATEGY

A weight-gain strategy is a change in eating habits designed to increase a person's weight. People who might need to develop a weight-gain strategy are those who have lost a lot of weight due to illness or an EATING DISORDER, those who are chronically UNDERWEIGHT due to a high rate of BODY METABOLISM, athletes and other active people who use up a great deal of energy through EXERCISE, and older people who have experienced a decline in APPETITE.

Two changes in eating habits are essential to any weight-gain strategy: increasing the proportion of high-calorie foods in the diet and simply eating larger quantities of food. A program of STRENGTH TRAINING will help convert gained pounds into muscle as well as fat. A sensible weight-gain strategy will put on pounds gradually. To gain 1 pound (0.45 kg) per week, you will need to add at least 500 calories per day to your diet.

Consuming More Calories If you need to increase your CALORIE intake, try to eat more high-calorie foods at meals. This, of course, is the opposite of the advice given to people who want to maintain their weight or lose weight. However, the foods highest in calories are often those highest in FATS. Too much fat, especially *saturated fat,* is bad for anyone because it leads to an increased risk of heart disease. To increase your calorie intake without adding too much fat, try consuming foods that pack a lot of CARBOHYDRATES and PROTEINS into a small space instead of filling you up with WATER and FIBER. Dried fruits and low-fat baked goods are examples. You can also increase your intake of *unsaturated fats,* which are not as harmful to health. Use a calorie chart to identify high-calorie foods that you find appealing.

HEALTHY CHOICES

Changing Eating Habits A change in the way you eat is also necessary if you begin consuming larger quantities. Instead of filling up on soups, beverages, or salads early in a meal, eat high-calorie foods first. Eat snacks between meals, but not so close to mealtime that they ruin your appetite for full-size meals. A high-calorie snack at bedtime can help. If you find that you cannot eat a large meal all at once, try eating several small meals throughout the day. Instead of drinking water, try juice, milk, or a high-calorie beverage such as a milk shake. If you still have trouble consuming enough calories, consider a high-calorie liquid supplement.

CONSULT A
PHYSICIAN

Cautions Anyone who has lost weight unexpectedly should consult a physician to be sure that the weight loss is not a symptom of a health problem that needs treatment. If you have always been thin, be aware that gaining weight may not be necessary. Being only a few pounds underweight poses no serious health problems. Still, many thin people would rather gain a few pounds, usually because they think that doing so would improve their appearance. Underweight people can gain weight safely by using nutritious foods to produce a slow, steady gain until the desired goal is reached. (See also FATS, OILS, AND SWEETS; WEIGHT ASSESSMENT; WEIGHT MANAGEMENT.)

▶ WEIGHT-LOSS STRATEGY

A weight-loss strategy is a change in lifestyle for the purpose of losing excess BODY FAT. Weight-loss strategies are usually followed by people who are OVERWEIGHT or obese. Losing weight can improve one's physical appearance and reduce the many health risks associated with excess weight.

Weight-loss strategies vary, depending on individual needs. Some are meant to be followed for only a short time in order to reach a goal: for example, to lose a small amount of excess weight gained during a temporary period of inactivity. Others call for a permanent change in eating habits. Some involve a minor reduction in food intake, whereas others offer a comprehensive plan of DIET and EXERCISE. Because there are so many choices, it helps to know what makes a weight-loss strategy effective.

Elements of an Effective Strategy Any weight-loss strategy is likely to involve a change in diet. In order to lose weight, a person should take in fewer CALORIES each day than the body will burn for energy. One pound (0.45 kg) of body fat results from about 3,500 excess calories. Eating 500 fewer calories' worth of food every day, therefore, will produce a loss of 1 pound per week. Weight loss tends to be faster at the beginning of a diet because a lot of water—not fat—is lost. Then the rate slows somewhat. In general, you should focus on nutritious low-calorie foods and limit your consumption of high-calorie foods, especially FATS, OILS, AND SWEETS.

Exercise can also significantly aid in weight loss. Developing a more active LIFESTYLE will cause you to burn more calories and make it easier to keep your weight down. AEROBIC EXERCISE (brisk walking, jogging, cycling) burns calories, whereas STRENGTH TRAINING can add muscle tissue that contributes to a higher rate of BODY METABOLISM. A combination of diet and exercise is usually suggested as the best way to lose weight. Regular exercise is particularly valuable as a way to maintain weight loss.

A change in eating habits will probably be needed in order for a weight-loss strategy to work well. A person who is overweight may have developed habits of overeating or of eating too many of the wrong kinds of foods. Breaking these habits can help such a person avoid regaining lost pounds. Problem eating habits vary, but helpful changes in behavior

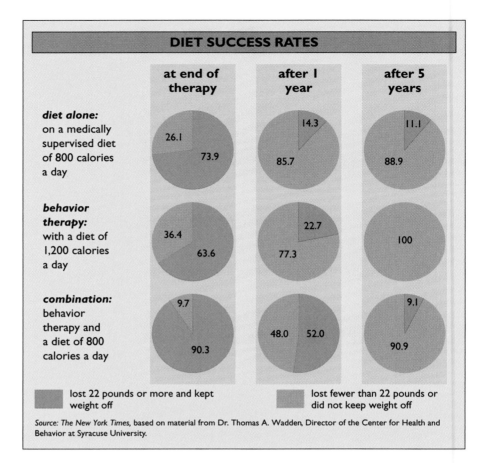

DIET SUCCESS RATES

	at end of therapy	after 1 year	after 5 years
diet alone: on a medically supervised diet of 800 calories a day	26.1 / 73.9	14.3 / 85.7	11.1 / 88.9
behavior therapy: with a diet of 1,200 calories a day	36.4 / 63.6	22.7 / 77.3	100
combination: behavior therapy and a diet of 800 calories a day	9.7 / 90.3	48.0 / 52.0	9.1 / 90.9

■ lost 22 pounds or more and kept weight off   ■ lost fewer than 22 pounds or did not keep weight off

Source: The New York Times, based on material from Dr. Thomas A. Wadden, Director of the Center for Health and Behavior at Syracuse University.

include eating more slowly, taking smaller portions of food, avoiding shopping for food when hungry, and eating regular meals.

CONSULT A PHYSICIAN

Medical professionals, such as your doctor or a *registered dietitian,* can offer useful advice about losing weight. They can help you decide whether or not to lose weight and, if so, how much. These professionals can also help you choose a safe, healthy, effective strategy. (See also NUTRITIONIST, **9.**)

There are many health benefits to be gained by losing extra pounds. Excess weight has been shown to increase the risks of disorders such as diabetes, high blood pressure, and heart disease. Lowering these risks can help people live longer and improve the quality of their lives.

Group weight-loss programs, such as Weight Watchers, are one popular way of losing weight. These groups offer support that many people find useful. The programs often provide information about nutrition. Most also use comprehensive plans that combine diet and exercise to help people achieve their goals. The long-term success rates of group programs and of other types of commercial programs and products are very low, however (see chart: Diet Success Rates).

Weight-Loss Strategies to Avoid Most nutritionists do not recommend losing excess weight too quickly. Doing so can cause health problems; in addition, weight that is lost quickly is often regained. There are many FAD DIETS that appeal to people's desire for a quick fix. Even when nutritionally sound, such diets can produce a steady pattern of losing and regaining pounds (sometimes called "yo-yo" dieting), rather than long-term weight loss. Experts suggest that a gradual loss of 1 to 2 pounds (0.45 to 1 kg) per week is safer and more effective than sudden loss or repeated dieting. It is a good idea to get medical advice before trying any diet that severely restricts the daily intake of calories.

Some people feel social pressure to lose weight. People who are not actually overweight sometimes attempt to lose weight anyway, which can cause serious health problems. (See also EATING DISORDERS.)

HEALTHY CHOICES
▪▪▪▪▪▪▪▪▪▪▪▪▪

Healthful Weight Loss   The best weight-loss strategy is one that will enable you to achieve and maintain a normal weight. Gradual weight loss resulting from a nutritious diet, good eating habits, and exercise is usually most successful. If you feel that you need to lose weight, first determine your goals. Then select a safe, effective, and long-lasting strategy to get the most satisfying results. (See also DIET AIDS; DIET FOOD; WEIGHT ASSESSMENT; WEIGHT MANAGEMENT.)

▶ WEIGHT MANAGEMENT

Weight management is the use of a diet and exercise program to maintain a healthy body weight. Successful weight management is achieved by combining proper NUTRITION with sensible eating and EXERCISE habits. For weight management to be effective, it must become part of a person's LIFESTYLE.

An important part of weight management involves managing BODY COMPOSITION, particularly the amount of fat in the body. The percentage of fat in a person's body affects his or her physical and social health. Being OVERWEIGHT or UNDERWEIGHT can reduce the body's stamina and increase risk for diseases such as heart disease and hypertension. In addition, a person's weight affects his or her self-image, self-esteem, and relationships with others.

How the Body Regulates Weight   The body maintains its weight when the amount of *food energy* taken in as CALORIES equals the amount

Weight Management. *An effective and healthful program of weight management takes body composition into consideration.*

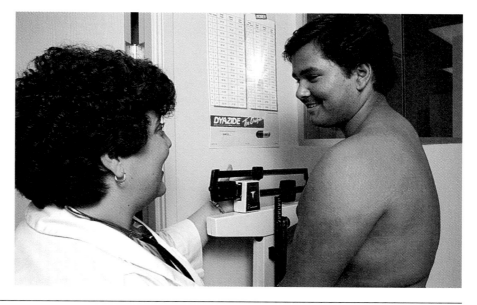

of *physical energy* expended in calories. When intake exceeds output, a person will gain weight. When output exceeds input, a person will lose weight. This relationship is called the *energy balance equation*.

The concept of weight management hinges on this balance. If people want to lose weight, they have to expend more calories than they consume, an essential element of any WEIGHT-LOSS STRATEGY. To gain weight, they have to take in more calories than they use as the basis of any WEIGHT-GAIN STRATEGY.

The key to weight management is to increase or decrease these variables depending on your current practices. To lose weight, you need to decrease your calorie intake, increase your physical activity, or both. A pound (0.45 kg) of fat tissue equals roughly 3,500 calories. For every pound you want to lose, you have to adjust your balance of energy so that you burn 3,500 calories more than you consume. To gain weight, you have to reverse the balance. For every pound you want to gain, you have to take in 3,500 calories more than you use. Moderate exercise will help convert the extra calories to muscle instead of fat.

To determine whether you need to lose weight, gain weight, or improve your body composition, you would need a WEIGHT ASSESSMENT. Ideally, this will take into account both your weight and your body composition.

Eating Right to Manage Weight To maintain your weight, you need to take in the same number of calories that you burn. However, calories from FATS are more easily converted to BODY FAT than those from other sources. Problems such as heart disease have also been linked to a high-fat diet. The best diet for weight management is therefore one that is low in fats and high in CARBOHYDRATES and contains all the other NUTRIENTS the body needs. Your diet should include plenty of whole grains, fresh fruits, and vegetables. Fatty foods that are high in calories and low in nutrients, such as FAST FOODS, fatty meats, and rich desserts, should be eaten only in moderation. A healthy diet should be a way of life, not just a short-term change.

HEALTHY CHOICES
● ● ● ● ● ● ● ● ● ● ● ● ●

Using Exercise to Manage Weight Exercise is essential to weight management and good health. Regular physical activity can help people lose weight and (depending on the activity) gain muscle. In addition to burning extra calories, it strengthens the heart and lungs and increases general well-being.

According to the American College of Sports Medicine, the best exercise program for weight management includes AEROBIC EXERCISE that is performed at least three times a week for a minimum of 20 minutes each time. However, even more important than the type or timing of exercise is making physical activity a regular part of your lifestyle. Because exercise must be both regular and consistent to be effective, people should choose activities they enjoy and are willing to continue on a routine basis throughout their lives. (See also DIETS; ENERGY, FOOD; ENERGY, PHYSICAL; RISK FACTORS.)

· ·

▶ **WELLNESS**

Wellness is a state of physical, mental, and emotional well-being. People achieve wellness by making behavior choices that enable them to enjoy life to the fullest.

Every day people make decisions that affect their health. They decide what to eat, how to spend their time, and with whom they will spend their time. On most days, they also decide how to cope with particular problems or how to plan for future needs. These and many other decisions contribute to an individual's LIFESTYLE. Wellness is achieved by making those lifestyle decisions that are best for overall health.

The concept of wellness is closely related to the idea of preventive medicine. In both cases, the focus is on making choices that reduce the risk of illness and enhance a person's physical, mental, and emotional well-being. (See also PREVENTIVE MEDICINE, **9**.)

► YOGA

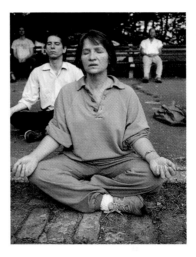

Yoga. *Yoga is popular among people of many ages and fitness levels. It can be an excellent way to relieve stress and even improve concentration.*

Yoga is a process that consists of assuming and holding a series of certain physical postures, called asanas. These postures are designed to enhance FLEXIBILITY and STRENGTH and relax the body. In addition, yoga involves breathing exercises, and many yoga instructors teach breathing control to help students achieve and sustain the asanas. Various styles of yoga exist; hatha yoga is the most popular in the United States and is the style discussed in this entry.

Practicing Yoga Although yoga includes numerous asanas, an effective exercise routine may be based on perhaps a dozen, with each person adding and varying postures over time. Yoga differs from most other forms of physical exercise in that the asanas involve only limited movement. A person assumes the different postures, holds them, and continues to breathe normally. Achieving the postures requires stretching, twisting , balancing, and bending.

Although many people practice yoga on their own, a variety of yoga classes are taught at FITNESS CENTERS and other community locations. Some classes combine yoga postures with other kinds of exercise or with meditation. Yoga classes may also have a spiritual component.

Benefits Practicing yoga on a regular basis offers a variety of benefits for both body and mind. Studies have shown that yoga can improve blood circulation and decrease HEART RATE. Yoga's physical movements help to loosen joints, relax muscles, and, over time, enhance muscle tone and posture. Yoga's breathing techniques can improve respiration and ease both physical and emotional tension. Some people also find that yoga increases their energy and enhances concentration.

SUPPLEMENTARY SOURCES

Brody, Jane. 1987. *Jane Brody's nutrition book*. New York: Bantam.

Clark, Nancy. 1997. *Nancy Clark's sports nutrition guidebook*. 2d ed. Champaign, Ill.: Human Kinetics.

Coleman, Ellen. 1997. *Eating for endurance*. 3d ed. Palo Alto, Calif.: Bull Publishing.

Copen, David, and Mark Rubenstein. 1987. *Heartplan: Complete program for total fitness of heart and mind*. New York: McGraw-Hill.

Duyff, Roberta Larson. 1998. *The American Dietetic Association's complete food and nutrition guide*. Minneapolis: Chronimed.

Eagles, Douglas A. 1987. *Nutritional diseases*. New York: Franklin Watts.

Glover, Bob, and Jack Shepherd. 1989. *The family fitness handbook*. New York: Penguin.

Horovitz, Emmanuel. 1990. *Cholesterol control made easy: How to lower your cholesterol for a healthier heart*. Los Angeles: Health Trend.

Kane, June K. 1990. *Coping with diet fads*. New York: Rosen Publishing Group.

Katch, Frank I., and William D. McArdle. 1993. *Introduction to nutrition, exercise, and health*. 4th ed. Philadelphia: Lea & Febiger.

Kettelkamp, Larry. 1986. *Modern sports science*. New York: William Morrow.

Kosich, Daniel. 1995. *Get real: A personal guide to real-life weight management*. San Diego: IDEA, International Association of Fitness Professionals.

Lee, Sally. 1990. *New theories on diet and nutrition*. New York: Franklin Watts.

Maloney, Michael, and Rachel Kranz. 1991. *Straight talk about eating disorders*. New York: Facts on File.

Mayer, Jean. 1990. *Dr. Jean Mayer's diet and nutrition guide*. New York: Pharos.

Quincy, Matthew. 1991. *Diet right! The consumer's guide to diet and weight loss programs*. Berkeley, Calif.: Conari.

Roth, Eli M., and Sandra L. Streicher. 1995. *Good cholesterol, bad cholesterol*. 2d ed. Rocklin, Calif.: Prima.

Sherman, Roberta T., and Ron A. Thompson. 1997. *Bulimia: A guide for family and friends*. San Francisco: Jossey-Bass.

Sleamaker, Rob. 1996. *Serious training for endurance athletes*. Champaign, Ill.: Human Kinetics.

Tracy, Lisa. 1985. *The gradual vegetarian*. New York: M. Evans.

ORGANIZATIONS

American Academy of Pediatrics
141 Northwest Point Boulevard
P.O. Box 927
Elk Grove Village, IL 60009
(847) 228-5005
(800) 433-9016
www.aap.org
kidsdocs@aap.org

American Anorexia/Bulimia Association
165 West 46th Street, Suite 1108
New York, NY 10036
(212) 575-6200
www.members.aol.com/amanbu
amanbu@aol.com

American Diabetes Association
1660 Duke Street
Alexandria, VA 22314
(800) 232-3472
www.diabetes.org

American Dietetic Association
216 West Jackson Boulevard
Suite 800
Chicago, IL 60606-6995
(312) 899-0040
www.eatright.org

American Heart Association
7272 Greenville Avenue
Dallas, TX 75231
(214) 373-6300
www.amhrt.org

American Running and Fitness Association
4405 East West Highway, Suite 405
Bethesda, MD 20814
(301) 913-9517
(800) 776-2732
www.arfa.org
arfa@aol.com

Asthma and Allergy Foundation of America
1125 Fifteenth Street, NW
Washington, DC 20036
(202) 466-7643
www.aafa.org

Center for Chronic Disease Prevention and Health Promotion
Centers for Disease Control and Prevention
1600 Clifton Road, NE
Atlanta, GA 30333
(404) 639-3311
www.cdc.gov
nesl@cdc.gov

Food and Drug Administration
Office of Consumer Affairs (HFE-88)
5600 Fishers Lane, (Room 16-85)
Rockville, MD 20857
(301) 827-4420
(800) 532-4440
www.fda.gov/oca/oca.htm

Institute of Medicine
Food and Nutrition Board
2101 Constitution Avenue, NW
Washington, DC 20418
(202) 334-2169
www.nas.edu/info

International Center for Sports Nutrition
502 South 44th Street, Suite 3012
Omaha, NE 68105
(402) 559-5505

Disabled Sports USA
451 Hungerford Drive, Suite 100
Rockville, MD 20850
(301) 217-0968
www.dsusa.org/tildendsusa/dsusa
dsusa@dsusa.org

Wheelchair Sports USA
3595 East Fountain Boulevard, Suite L-1
Colorado Springs, CO 80910
(719) 574-1150
www.wsusa.org
wsusa@abl.com

Office of Disease Prevention and Health
Promotion
National Health Information Center
P.O. Box 1133
Washington, DC 20013
(800) 336-4797
(301) 565-4167 (in Maryland)
nhic-nt.health.org
nhicinfo@health.org

President's Council on Physical Fitness
and Sports
701 Pennsylvania Avenue, NW, Suite 250
Washington, DC 20004
(202) 272-3421
phs.os.dhhs.gov/progorg/ophs/pcpfs.htm

Special Olympics International
1325 G Street, NW, Suite 500
Washington, DC 20005
(202) 628-3630
www.specialolympics.org
soimail@aol.com

INDEX

Italicized page numbers refer to illustrations or charts.

Abrasions, 107
Acesulfame-K (Sunett), 9
Acupuncture, 110
Additives, food, 59–60
Adequate intakes (AIs), 21–22, 84, 98, 124, 126
Adrenaline, basal metabolic rate and, 18
Aerobic dance, *4, 4. See also* Aerobic exercise;
    Endurance; Fitness training; Flexibility;
    Heart rate
Aerobic exercise, 4–6, 45
    endurance and, 39, 40, 58
    fitness and, 56
    fitness training and, 58
    training for sports and, 106
    for weight management, 140
    See also Cycling; Flexibility; Running;
        Sports and fitness; Strength; Swimming;
        Walking
Aerobics and Fitness Association of America, 57
Age, basal metabolic rate and, 18
Agricultural chemicals, 6–7, 91. *See also* Food
    additives; Food safety
Alcoholics, malnutrition among, 80
Allergies, food, *60,* 60–61
American College of Sports Medicine, 57, 93,
    140
American Council on Exercise, 93
American Diabetes Association, 36
American Heart Association, 93, 104
Amino acids, 15, 20, 81, 96, 121
Amphetamine, 30
Anabolic steroids, 13
Anabolism, 17
Anaerobic exercise, *5, 7,* 7–8, 45. *See also*
    Aerobic exercise; Endurance; Fitness; Fitness
    training; Strength training
Anaphylactic shock, food allergy and, 61
Anemia, 76, 79, 87, 124, 125, 127
Anorexia, 37–38, *38*
Anorexia nervosa, 8
Antibodies in breast milk, 21
Antimicrobials, 59
Antioxidants, 10, 59, 125, 127
Appetite, 8, 74. *See also* Diets; Eating disorders;
    Food craving; Hunger; Weight management
Appetite suppressants, 8, 30
Artificial sweeteners, 9, 12, 59. *See also* Diet
    foods; Sugar
Asanas (yoga), 141
Ascorbic acid. *See* Vitamin C
Aspartame, 9
Atherosclerosis, cholesterol and, 26
Athletes, diets for, 36
Athletic footwear, 9–10, 101, 109
Atrophy, 112
Attitudes, health and, 77

Back pain and injuries, 106–7, *107*
Bacterial contamination, 69

Bacterial foodborne illnesses, 61–62
Balanced diet, 11
    breakfast as part of, 20
    Food Guide Pyramid and, 64–65
    vegetarian, 120–21
Balance in strength training, 113
Ballistic stretching, 115
Basal metabolic rate, 18, *42, 42*
Beans, 80
Behavior patterns, 77
Beriberi, 123
Beta carotene, 10, 71, 122, 123. *See also*
    Nutrients; Vitamins
Beverages, 10–12, 132
BHT, 59
Bicycle riding. *See* Cycling
Bile, 26
Binge eating, 38, 39
Bioelectrical impedance, 15, 135
Biofeedback, 99
Bioflavonoids, 125
Biotechnology, 71
Biotin, *124,* 124, *130*
Bland diet, 36
Blisters, sports and, 107
Blood, 132
Blood proteins, 97
Blood sugar level, 73. *See also* Glucose
Bodybuilding, *13,* 13–14. *See also* Anaerobic
    exercise; Strength training
Body composition, 14–15
    body building and changing, 13
    fitness and, 57
    managing, 139
    measuring, 15
    weight assessment and, 133
    See also Diets; Eating disorders; Obesity
Body fat, 14–15, 15–16, 17, 41. *See also* Body
    composition; Cholesterol; Energy, food; Fats,
    oils, and sweets group; Risk factors
Body image, 38, 134
Body-mass index (BMI), 15, *16,* 16–17, 92, 134
Body metabolism, 17–19
    fasting and, 50–51
    measuring, 18
    overweight and, 92
    protein and, 97
    See also Digestion; Nutrients
Body temperature
    basal metabolic rate and, 18
    exercise and heat injury, 46, 47
Body types, *14*
Bomb calorimeter, 23
Bone strength, 56
Botulism, 59, 62, 70
Bran, 19
Bread, cereal, rice, and pasta group, 19–20, 65.
    See also Exchange system; Food Guide
    Pyramid; Starch

Breakfast, 20–21
Breast-feeding, 21
Breast milk, 21
Breathing exercises, 99, 141
Brown rice, 19
Brown sugar, 117
Bruises, 107
Bulimia, 30, 37, 38–39
Butterfat, 83

Caffeine, 12, 13
Calcium, 21–22, 83, 84, *86,* 121. *See also*
    Minerals; Vitamins
Calcium deficiency, 22
Calcium phosphate, 21
Calcium propionate, 59
Calcium supplements, 33
Calisthenics, 114
Calorie(s), 23–24
    diet and supply of, 34
    energy-balance equation, 23, 41, 140
    in fats, 53
    measuring food energy by, 41
    requirements for energy, *42, 42*
    to support basal metabolism, 18
    weight-gain strategy and, 136
    weight-loss strategy and, 137
    weight management and, 139–40
    See also Body metabolism; Diets
Campylobacter jejuni, 62
Canning, 67–68, 70
Carbohydrate loading, 25, 111
Carbohydrates, 24–25, 40, 88–89, *89*
    complex, 24, *25,* 25, 111–12
    craving for foods high in, 63
    simple, 24, *25,* 112
    See also Bread, cereal, rice, and pasta
        group; Energy, food; Fiber; Fruit group;
        Glucose; Nutrients; Starch; Sugar
Cardiovascular endurance, 39, *39,* 56, 104
Cardiovascular fitness, 4, 5, 6, 74, 100
Catabolism, 17
Catalyst, water as, 132
Celiac disease, diet for, 36
Cereals, 19
Chafing, 107
Chemical preservation, 59, 68
Chemicals, agricultural, 6–7, 91
Children, malnutrition among, 79
Chiropractors, 109
Chloride, 86
Cholesterol, 5, 26–27, *27,* 53, 54, 81, 83. *See
    also* Body fat; Fast food; Food labeling; Meat,
    poultry, fish, dry beans, eggs, and nuts group;
    Obesity; Risk factors
Chromium, 84, 87, 88
Circuit training, 114
Cleanliness, food preparation and, 70
Clostridium botulinum, 62

Clostridium perfringens, 61
Coffee, 13
Cold method of food preservation, 68
Coloring agents, 60
Colostrum, 21
Complementary proteins, 81
Complete proteins, 81, 96
Complex carbohydrates, 24, *25,* 25, 111–12
Compulsive overeating, 39
Concussion, 107
Contamination of food, 69–70
Contract-relax stretching, 115
Cooldown exercise, 131, 132
Copper, *87,* 87
Cows' milk, sensitivity to, 60
Cramps, 107
    heat, 46
Crash diets, 49
Craving, food, 63–64
Cream, 83
Creatine, 14
Cross-country ski machines, 48
Cross training, 27–28. *See also* Aerobic exercise;
    Exercise; Fitness; Fitness training; Sports and
    fitness; Strength training
Cryptosporidium, 62
Cultured milk products, 83
Cured foods, 68
Cyclamate, 9
Cycling, 28–29
    on stationary bicycles, 47–48, *48*
    See also Fitness; Fitness training; Heart
    rate
Cyclospora cayetanesis parasite, 62

Daily Values, 66
Dairy products. *See* Milk, yogurt, and cheese
    group
Dance, aerobic, 4
Dark green leafy vegetables, 119
Deep yellow vegetables, 119
Dehydration, *29,* 29–30, 111, 133
    heat exhaustion and, 46
    perspiration and, 29
    See also Beverages; Exercise and heat in-
    jury
Dexfenfluramine (Redux), 30
Dextrose. *See* Glucose
Diabetes mellitus, 26
    malnutrition and, 79
Diabetic diet, 36
Diarrhea
    dehydration and, 29, 133
    traveler's, 62
Diet aids, 30–31. *See also* Appetite; Calorie(s);
    Dietary guidelines; Diets; Exercise; Fad diets;
    Fiber; Lifestyle; Liposuction; Nutrition;
    Obesity; Weight-loss strategy; Weight man-
    agement
Dietary guidelines, 31–32, *32,* 53, 65. *See also*
    Adequate intakes (AIs); Calorie(s);
    Cholesterol; Recommended dietary al-
    lowance (RDA); Nutrition; Nutrients;
    Weight management
Dietary reference intakes (DRIs), 86, 98,
    128–29, *130*
Dietary supplements, 33
Dietetics, 91

Diet foods, 31, 33–34, 102. *See also* Appetite;
    Calorie(s); Diet aids; Dietary guidelines;
    Diets; Fats; Food labeling; Obesity; Weight-
    loss strategy; Weight management
Dietitians, 44, 91
Diet pills, 30
Diets, 34–36
    carbohydrates in, 25
    as controllable risk factor, 100
    controlling cholesterol with, 27
    elements of healthy, 34–35
    exchange system for planning, 43–44
    malnutrition caused by deficiencies in,
    78–79
    to treat and prevent illness, 36
    types of, 35–36, 49–50, 104
    water in, 132
    weight assessment and, 136
    for weight management, 140
    See also Appetite; Balanced diet; Diet
    foods; Dietary guidelines; Fad diets;
    Fiber; Nutrition; Phytochemicals;
    Vegetarian diet
Diet success rate, *138*
Digestion, 36–37, 60. *See also* Appetite; Body
    metabolism; Energy, food; Hunger
Digestive system, processes of, 37
Disaccharide, 116, 117
Disease, malnutrition caused by, 79
Diuretics, 12, 30, 104
Drying, food preservation by, 67

Eating disorders, 8, 37–39, 79. *See also*
    Fasting; Food craving; Malnutrition;
    Underweight; Weight assessment
Edema, 133
Eggs, 80
    Salmonella contamination of, 70
Elderly, malnutrition among the, 79
Electric conductivity, 15, 135
Electrolyte, 102
Emulsifiers, 60
Endurance, 39–40, 56
    aerobic exercise for, 39, 40, 58
    cardiovascular, *39,* 39, 56, 104
    cross training for, 27
    energy needs for, 111
    muscular, 27, 39, 40, 56, 104, *105,* 105
    See also Exercise; Fitness; Strength training
Energy, food, 15, *40,* 40–41
    athletes' needs, 110–11
    energy-balance equation, 23, 41, 140
    See also Body metabolism; Calorie(s);
    Energy, physical; Nutrients; Weight
    management
Energy, physical, 41–42, *42. See also* Energy,
    food; Exercise; Nutrients; Rest; Weight man-
    agement
Energy-balance equation, 23, 41, 140
Enriched breads, 19
Enriched foods, 59, 123
    breads, 19
Enzymes, 87
    food spoilage and, 67
    muscular endurance and, 40
Ephedrine (ma huang), 8, 30
Ergometers, 48
Escherichia coli, diarrhea from, 62

Essential amino acids, 81, 96
Exchange system, 42–44. *See also* Dietary
    guidelines; Food Guide Pyramid
Exercise, 44–45
    body composition and, 14
    calories and energy expenditure in, 23
    cross training, 27–28
    fitness and, 56–57
    fluid replacement during, *29*
    forms of, 44–45
    health and, 44
    interval training, 75
    lifestyle and, 45
    metabolic rate and, *17,* 18
    overweight and, 92
    personal trainer and, 93
    precautions about, 45
    relaxation after, 99
    risk factors based on, 100
    warm-up and cooldown, 131–32
    weight-loss strategy and, 35, 137
    weight management and, 140
    See also Aerobic dance; Aerobic exercise;
    Anaerobic exercise; Energy, physical;
    Exercise and heat injury; Exercise ma-
    chines; Fitness training; Risk factors;
    Sports and fitness; Sports injuries;
    Sports medicine; Strength training;
    Walking
Exercise and heat injury, *46,* 46–47. *See also*
    Dehydration; Exercise; Perspiration
Exercise machines, 47–49, 57, 114. *See also*
    Cross training; Endurance; Fitness training;
    Strength training

Fad diets, 49–50, 138–39. *See also* Diet aids;
    Diets; Fasting; Malnutrition; Obesity;
    Weight management
Fast food, *50,* 50. *See also* Fats, oils, and sweets
    group; Junk food
Fasting, 50–51. *See also* Fad diets; Weight-loss
    strategy
Fat, body. *See* Body fat
Fat cells, 16
Fatfold test, 15. *See also* Skinfold measurement
Fatigue, 51–52. *See also* Malnutrition
Fats, 52, 52–53, *89,* 89
    in fast foods, 50
    low-fat diet, 36
    in meat, poultry, fish, dry beans, eggs, and
    nuts group, 81
    saturated, 27, *27,* 52, 53, 54, 81, 83, 136
    unsaturated, 52, 53, 136
    vegetarian diet and, 122
    weight-gain strategy and, 136
    See also Body fat; Carbohydrates; Energy,
    food; Fats, oils, and sweets group;
    Nutrients; Obesity; Proteins
Fats, oils, and sweets group, *54,* 54, 65. *See also*
    Dietary guidelines; Exchange system
Fat-soluble vitamins, 123, 126, 127, 128,
    129–30
Fatty acids, 15–16, 41
FD&C Red No. 40, 60
Female athlete triad, 119
Fenfluramine (Pondimin), 30
Fertilizers, 6–7, 91
Fiber, 24, *55,* 55–56

low- and high-fiber diets, 36
vegetarian diet and, 122
See also Carbohydrates; Dietary guidelines
Fish, 80
Fitness, 56–57
body metabolism and, 18–19
cardiovascular, 4, 5, 6, 74, 100
President's Council on Physical Fitness and Sports, 95
swimming for, 117–18
See also Aerobic exercise; Body composition; Endurance; Flexibility; Sports and fitness; Strength; Walking; Weight assessment
Fitness center, 57, 57
Fitness training, 57–58. *See also* Cross training; Energy, physical; Sports and fitness
Flat breads, 19
Flavoring agents, 59. *See also* Artificial sweeteners; Monosodium glutamate (MSG)
Flexibility, 13, 58–59, 105
fitness and, 56–57
See also Fitness training; Sports injuries; Strength training
Fluoride, 84, 86, 88
Folate, 20, 124, 124, 130
Folic acid, 20, 124
Folk medicine, 94
Food additives, 59–60. *See also* Food allergies and intolerances; Food labeling; Food preservation methods; Food safety; Organic food
Food allergies and intolerances, 60, 60–61, 72
Food and Drug Administration (FDA), 7, 8, 30, 33, 34, 59, 60, 67, 68
Food and Nutrition Board of the National Academy of Sciences, 84, 98, 128
Foodborne illness, 51–53, 69, 70. *See also* Food safety
Food craving, 63, 63–64. *See also* Appetite; Weight management
Food energy. *See* Energy, food
Food Guide Pyramid, 64, 64–65
balanced diet and, 11
bread, cereal, rice, and pasta in, 20
exchange system guidelines vs., 43
fats, oils, and sweets in, 54–56
fruits in, 71
meat, poultry, fish, dry beans, eggs, and nuts in, 82
milk, yogurt, and cheese in, 83–84
vegetables in, 119–20
See also Dietary guidelines; Exchange system; Nutrients
Food labeling, 64–67
for diet foods, 33–34
for organic foods, 92
RDAs and, 66, 98
for snack foods, 102
for sodium, 104
See also Dietary guidelines
Food Marketing Institute, 50
Food preservation methods, 59, 60, 67–68. *See also* Food safety
Food product dating, 67
Food safety, 63, 68–70. *See also* Food allergies and intolerances; Food labeling
Food spoilage, 67
Foot injuries, 107, 108

Fortified foods, 59
cereals, 19
Free radicals, 10, 125, 127
Free weights, 49, 114
Freeze-drying, 68
Freezing method of preserving foods, 68
Fructose, 71, 116–17
Fruitarian diet, 120
Fruit drinks, 12–13
Fruit group, 70–71, 71. *See also* Dietary guidelines; Exchange system; Food Guide Pyramid

Galactose, 117
Genetically engineered food, 71–72
Glucagon, 73
Glucose, 15, 20, 40, 41, 72, 72–73, 110, 112, 116. *See also* Body metabolism; Digestion; Energy, food; Energy, physical
Gluten-free diet, 36
Glycogen, 7, 15, 41, 72, 110
Goiter, 87, 102
Gout, low-purine diet for, 36
Grains. *See* Bread, cereal, rice, and pasta group
Group weight-loss programs, 138
Growth regulators, 7

HDL cholesterol, 5, 26
Head injuries, 107
Health club. *See* Fitness center
Healthy Eating Index, 32
Heart, strength of, 56
Heart disease, excess body fat and, 16
Heart rate, 5, 73–74
circuit training and, 114
target range, 6, 74
See also Aerobic exercise; Fitness; Fitness training; Running; Sports and fitness
Heat cramps, 46
Heat exhaustion, 46
Heatstroke, 46–47
Height and weight chart, 134, 135
Heme iron, 76
Hemoglobin, iron in, 75
Hepatitis, 62
Herbal supplements, 33
Herbal teas, 13
Heredity and environment, risk factors involving, 100
High-density lipoprotein (HDL), 26
HDL cholesterol, 5, 26
High-fiber diet, 36
Histamines, 60
Homogenization, 83
Honey, 117
Hormones
body metabolism and, 17, 18
calcium level and, 21
cholesterol and, 26
growth regulators mimicking, 7
thyroid, 87
Hunger, 8, 74–75
Hydrogenation, 53
Hydrostatic weighing, 15, 135
Hyperglycemia, 73
Hypertension, 85
sodium in diet and, 102, 104
Hypoglycemia, 73
Hypothalamus, sense of hunger and, 75

Hypothermia, 118
Hypothyroidism, 26

Incomplete proteins, 81, 96
Ingredients, list of, 65–66
Injuries. *See* Sports injuries
Insecticides, food contamination by, 62
Insects, food contamination by, 70
Insoluble fibers, 55
Insoluble proteins, 96–97
Insulin, blood sugar level and, 73
Interval training, 75
Iodine, 84, 85, 87, 102
Iron, 75–76, 85, 86–87
Iron deficiency, 76, 121
Iron-deficiency anemia, 76
Irradiation, 68
Isoflavones, 94
Isokinetic exercise, 114
Isometric exercise, 113
Isothiocyanates, 94
Isotonic exercise, 114

Juices, 12–13
Junk food, 102

Kidneys, 132
Kilocalorie, 23
Knee injuries, 107, 108
Kwashiorkor, 79

Labeling, food. *See* Food labeling
Lacerations, 107
Lactase, 60
Lactic acid, 7
Lacto-ovovegetarians, 120, 121
Lactose, 117
Lactose intolerance, 60, 83, 117
Lactovegetarians, 120, 121
Lanugo, 38
Lap, swimming a, 117
Laxatives, 30, 103
LDL cholesterol, 26, 27
Legumes, 80, 112, 119
Length, swimming a, 117
Lifestyle, 77, 77–78
as controllable risk factor, 100
digestion and, 37
exercise and, 45
fatigue and, 51
weight management and, 139
wellness and, 141
See also Diets; Rest
Limonene, 94
Lipids, 15–16
Lipoproteins, 26
Liposuction, 31. *See also* Body composition
Liquid diets, 49
Listeria monocytogenes, 62
Listeriosis, 62
Low-density lipoprotein (LDL), 26
LDL cholesterol, 26, 27
Low-fat diet, 36
Low-fiber diet, 36
Low-impact aerobics, 6
Low-purine diet, 36
Low-sodium diet, 36, 104
Lungs, aerobic exercise and, 5
Lymph, 132

Macrobiotic diet, 120
Macrominerals, 84
Macronutrients, 24, 52, 88–89, *89*, 95. *See also*
    Carbohydrates; Fats; Proteins
Magnesium, 85–86, *86*
Ma huang (ephedrine), 8, 30
Malnutrition, 78–80, 90, 97. *See also* Anemia;
    Eating disorders; Nutrition; Underweight
Mammary glands, 21
Manganese, 84, *87*, 87–88
Maple syrup, 117
Marasmus, 79
Marathons, 100
Maximum heart rate, 74
Meat, poultry, fish, dry beans, eggs, and nuts
    group, 80–82. *See also* Dietary guidelines;
    Exchange system
Meat thermometer, using, *69*, 69
Meditation, 99
Melatonin, 33
Menopause, 22
Menstrual cycle, cravings during, 63
Metabolism, 40
    yo-yo syndrome and metabolic rate, 49
    See also Body metabolism
Microminerals, 84
Micronutrients, 88, *89*, 89. *See also* Minerals;
    Vitamins
Microorganisms, food spoilage and, 67
Milk, breast, 21
Milk, yogurt, and cheese group, 13, 82–84. *See
    also* Dietary guidelines; Exchange system
Minerals, 33, 71, 81, 83, 84–88, *85*, *86*, *87*, *89*,
    89. *See also* Body metabolism; Calcium; Iron;
    Nutrients; Potassium; Sodium; Vitamins
Molasses, 117
Molybdenum, 84, *87*, 88
Monosaccharide, 112, 116, 117
Monosodium glutamate (MSG), 59, 60, 103.
    See also Food additives; Salt
Monounsaturated fats, 27, *52*, 53
MSG, 59, 60, 103
Muscles
    aerobic exercise and, 5
    body building and, 13–14
Muscle strength, 56
Muscular endurance, 27, 39, 40, 56, 104, *105*,
    105
Myoglobin, 75

National Academy of Sports Medicine, 93
National Cancer Institute, 10, 94
Natural food. *See* Organic food
Nervous system, proteins and regulation of, 97
Neuritis, 124
Niacin, *124*, 124, *130*
Nitrites, 59
Nonfat dry milk, 83
Nonheme iron, 76
Nutrients, 88–89, *89*
    added to foods, 59
    from bread, cereal, rice, and pasta group, 20
    from breast milk, 21
    diet and supply of, 34–35
    digestion and, 37
    from fruits, 71
    from meat, poultry, fish, dry beans, eggs,
        and nuts group, 81

from milk, yogurt, and cheese, 82–83
RDA of, 97–98, *129*, *130*
from vegetables, 119
See also Carbohydrates; Fats; Minerals;
    Proteins; Vitamins; Water
Nutrition, 90–91
    sports, 110–11
    See also Body metabolism; Malnutrition;
        Nutrients; Phytochemicals
Nutritional therapy, 91
Nutrition Facts, 66
Nutritionists, 90–91
Nutrition labeling, *66*, 66
Nuts, 80

Obesity, 44, 54, 90, 92, 137
Oils. *See* Fats, oils, and sweets group
Olestra, 34
Onions, benefits of, 94
Organic food, 68, 91–92. *See also* Agricultural
    chemicals; Food safety
Organ meats, 80
Orthopedists, 109
Orthotic devices, 10, 101, 109
Osteomalacia, 126
Osteopathic physicians, 109
Osteoporosis, 22, 84, 113, 131
Overload, 45, 58, 113
Overweight, 92–93. *See also* Body metabolism;
    Diet aids; Diet foods; Diets; Obesity; Risk fac-
    tors; Weight assessment; Weight-loss strat-
    egy; Weight management
Oxygen debt, 7

Pancreas, blood sugar level and, 73
Pantothenic acid, *124*, 124, *130*
Parasites, foods contaminated by, 62
Pasta, 19–20
Pasteurization, 67, 83
Perceived exertion, rate of, 74
Perishable foods, 70
Perspiration, 29, 46, 47. *See also* Beverages;
    Dehydration; Exercise and heat injury
Pesticides, 7, 62, 91
Phenylketonuria, 9
Phenylpropanolamine, 30
Phosphorus, 84, *85*, *86*
Physical Activity and Health (Surgeon General),
    44
Physical energy. *See* Energy, physical
Physiological cravings, 63
Phytochemicals, 93–94. *See also* Beta carotene;
    Fiber; Minerals; Vitamin B complex; Vitamin
    C; Vitamin E
Pickling, 68
Podiatrists, 109
Polysaccharides, 111
Polyunsaturated fats, *53*, 53
Potassium, 84, 94–95, *95*. *See also* Minerals;
    Sodium
Potassium sorbate, 59
Poultry, 80
Poverty, malnutrition and, 79
Pregnancy, cravings during, 63
Preservatives, 59, 60, 67–68
President's Council on Physical Fitness and
    Sports, 95. *See also* Exercise; Fitness training;
    Sports and fitness

Preventive medicine, 141
Processed meats, 80
Progression in strength training, 113
Progressive muscle relaxation, 99
Pronation, 10, 101
Protein-calorie malnutrition, 79
Protein complementing, 96
Proteins, 81, 95–97, *96*
    athletes' needs for, 111
    as macronutrient, *89*, 89, 95
Psychological cravings, *63*, 63–64
Pulse, taking a, 74
Pyridoxine (B$_6$), *124*, 124, *130*

Quick breads, 19

Range of motion, 56, 58–59
Recommended dietary allowance (RDA), 97–98
    dietary supplements containing, 33
    on food labels, 66, 98
    of minerals, 84, 85
    of vitamins, 128, *129*
    See also Dietary guidelines
Refrigeration, 68
Registered dietitian, 91, 138
Regulation
    of dietary supplements, 33
    of food labeling, 33–34, 67
    See also Food and Drug Administration
        (FDA); U.S. Department of Agriculture
        (USDA)
Relaxation, 98–99
Resistance equipment, 49
Rest, 98–99. *See also* Energy, physical; Fatigue;
    Lifestyle
Resting heart rate, 74
Retinol. *See* Vitamin A
Riboflavin, *124*, 124, *130*
Rice, 19
RICE (Rest, Ice, Compress, Elevate), 106
Rickets, 22, 126
Risk factors, 99–100
Rodents, food contamination by, 70
Roughage. *See* Fiber
Running, 27, 100–101. *See also* Aerobic exer-
    cise; Body composition; Endurance; Fitness;
    Heart rate; Sports injuries

Saccharin, 9
Safety
    cycling, 29
    food, 63, 68–70
    running, 101
    strength training, 114
    swimming, 118
    walking, 131
Salmonella bacteria, 61–62, 70
Salt, 101–2, 103
    cravings for, 63
    low-sodium diet, 36, 104
    as preservative, 59, 68
    See also Minerals; Monosodium glutamate
        (MSG); Potassium
Satiety, 8, 75
Saturated fats, 27, *27*, *52*, 53, 54, 81, 83, 136
Scurvy, 125
Sedatives, 103
Sedentary lifestyle, 77

Seeds, 80
Selenium, 84, *85*, 88
Semivegetarians, 120
Set-point theory of weight, 18
Shellfish, 80
Shigellosis, 62
Shinsplints, 107, *108*
Simple carbohydrates, 24, *25*, 112
Skim milk, 83
Skinfold measurement, 15, *134, 135*
Snacking, 102–3. *See also* Fast food; Weight management
Sodium, 85, 94, *103*, 103–4. *See also* Calcium; Potassium; Vitamins; Water
Sodium bicarbonate (baking soda), 103
Sodium chloride. *See* Salt
Sodium nitrite, 59
Soluble fiber, 55
Soluble proteins, 97
Sorbic acid, 59
Sore muscles, 107
Sports and fitness, 104–6, *105*
    athletic footwear for, 9–10
    calories burned in various activities, *42*
    choosing a sport, 104–5
    training for sports, 106
    See also Endurance; Fitness training; Flexibility; Sports injuries; Strength
Sports injuries, 28, 106–9, *108*
    heat injury, 46–47
    preventing, 108–9, *110*, 110
    treating common types of, 106–8
    See also Athletic footwear; Sports medicine; Strength training; Stretching exercise
Sports medicine, 109–10, *110. See also* Sports injuries
Sports nutrition, 110–11
Sports psychologists, 110
Sprains and strains, sports and, 107, *108*
Stamina. *See* Endurance
Staphylococcus aureus, foodborne illness caused by, 61
Starch, 24, 111–12. *See also* Bread, cereal, rice, and pasta group; Carbohydrates; Energy, food; Nutrients
Starchy vegetables, 119
Static stretching, *115*, 115
Stationary bicycles, 47–48, *48*
Sterilization, 67
Steroids, anabolic, 13
Stimulants, 30
Strength, 8, 56, *105*, 106, 112–13, *113. See also* Exercise; Fitness; Strength training
Strength training, 13, 58, 106, 113–15, *114*.
    See also Bodybuilding; Endurance; Fitness; Strength
Stress, 77
    relaxation to reduce, 99
Stress test, 45
Stretching exercise, 45, 106, *115*, 115–16
    for flexibility, 58, 59
    See also Aerobic dance; Fitness; Running
Sucralose (Splenda), 9
Sucrose, 9, 117
Sugar, 116–17
    as food preservative, 68
    as preservative, 59

as simple carbohydrate, 24
    in soft drinks, 12
    See also Artificial sweeteners; Carbohydrates; Energy, food; Fats, oils, and sweets group; Fiber; Overweight; Starch
Supination, 10, 101
Surgeon General, 44
Surgery, weight loss through, 31
Sweets. *See* Fats, oils, and sweets group
Swimming, 27, 117–18

Target heart rate, 6, 74
Tartrazine, 60
Tea, 13
Temperature, basal metabolic rate and, 18
Tendinitis, sports and, *108,* 108
Thiamine, 123, *124, 130*
Thirst, 29–30, 133
    heat-related sports problems and, 47
Thyroid gland, overactive, 8
Thyroid hormones, 87
Thyroxine, 30
Toxins, 120
Toxoplasmosis, 62
Trace minerals, 84
Trainer, personal, 93
Training
    cross, 27–28
    endurance, 40
    fitness, 57–58
    interval, 75
    for sports, 106
    strength, 13, 58, 106, 113–15, *114*
Traveler's diarrhea, 62
Treadmills, 48–49
Tryptophan, 124

Ultrapasteurization, 67
Underweight, 118–19. *See also* Weight assessment; Weight-gain strategy
U.S. Department of Agriculture (USDA), 10, 31, 32, 64, 65, 70, 92
    Research Center on Aging, 94
U.S. Department of Health and Human Services, 31
Unsaturated fats, *52,* 53, 136
Urine, 132

Vegans, 35, 120–21
Vegetable group, 65, *119,* 119–20
Vegetarian diet, 35, 120–22, *121. See also* Diets; Vitamin B complex
Vitamin A, 10, 71, *122,* 122–23, 129
Vitamin A deficiency, 123
Vitamin B$_{12}$, 120–21, *124,* 124, *130*
Vitamin B$_6$, *124,* 124, *130*
Vitamin B complex, 123–24, *124*
    in diets for athletes, 36
Vitamin C, 59, 71, *125,* 125–26, *129*
    deficiency, 125
    See also Vitamin E
Vitamin D, 121, 126–27, *130*
    calcium level and, 21
    cholesterol and, 26
    deficiency, 126–27
Vitamin E, 59, *127,* 127, *129. See also* Vitamin C
Vitamin K, 127–28, *128, 129*

Vitamins, 33, *89,* 89, 128–30, *129, 130*
    fat-soluble, 123, 126, 127, 128, 129–30
    in fruits, 71
    in milk, 83
    RDAs for, 128, *129*
    water-soluble, 123, 125, 128
Vomiting
    bulimia and, 38
    dehydration and, 29, 133

Waist-to-hip ratio, 134
Walking, 131. *See also* Athletic footwear; Endurance
Warm-up and cooldown, 131–32
Water, 12, 132–33, *133*
    balance of, 133
    fluid needs/replacement during sports, 47, 111
    foods with high water content, 132, *133*
    See also Beverages; Body metabolism; Dehydration; Minerals
Water-soluble vitamins, 123, 125, 128
Weight assessment, 133–36, *134*
    body mass index and, 16–17
    methods of, 134–36
    See also Body composition; Diets; Eating disorders; Fitness; Obesity; Overweight; Underweight; Weight-gain strategy; Weight-loss strategy
Weight-gain strategy, 35, 119, 136–37. *See also* Body metabolism; Fats, oils, and sweets group; Underweight; Weight assessment; Weight management
Weight lifting, 8, 114. *See also* Strength training
Weight-loss strategy, 137–39
    diet foods for, 31, 33–34
    diets for, 35
    diet success rates, *138*
    elements of effective, 35, 137–38
    fad diets and, 49–50, 138–39
    for overweight, 93, 137–39
    running, 100–101
    strategies to avoid, 138–39
    to treat obesity, 137
    See also Diet aids; Weight assessment; Weight management
Weight machines, 49
Weight management, *139,* 139–40
    body metabolism and, 18
    eating right for, 140
    energy-balance equation and, 24, 41, 140
    excess body fat and, 15
    exercise for, 140
    See also Diets; Energy, food; Energy, physical; Lifestyle; Risk factors
Wellness, 140–41
White rice, 19
Whole-food diet, 120
Whole-grain breads, 19
Whole milk, 83

Yeast, 19
Yeast breads, 19
Yin and yang, 120
Yoga, *141,* 141
Yo-yo syndrome, 49, 139

Zinc, 84, *85,* 87